Psychiatric Mental Health Nursing
Made Easy

Beginner's Guide to Mental Health Nursing

Thorne James Blackwood

Psychiatric Mental Health Nursing

Made Easy

ISBN- 978-1-923238-62-6

Jstone Publishing

Preface

Welcome to " Psychiatric Mental Health Nursing Made Easy," a guide designed to demystify the complexities of mental health nursing and make accessible the essential practices and theories that underpin this crucial field. This book is intended for a wide audience—nursing students embarking on their careers, practicing nurses seeking to enhance their knowledge in mental health, and anyone interested in the vital work of mental health care.

The journey into mental health nursing is not just about acquiring knowledge; it's about developing a deep understanding of human behavior, mastering practical skills to manage diverse challenges, and cultivating compassion and empathy towards those in need. Mental health nursing is both an art and a science, requiring a delicate balance of technical skills and interpersonal acumen.

Why This Book?

Throughout my years of experience in both practicing and teaching mental health nursing, I've encountered numerous individuals overwhelmed by the intricacies of mental health conditions and the nuances of care required. This observation sparked the idea for a resource that could simplify complex concepts and offer practical guidance. "Mental Health Nursing Made Easy" aims to fill this gap by providing a clear, concise, and engaging exploration of mental health nursing.

What to Expect

The book is structured to guide you through the fundamentals of mental health nursing, starting with basic concepts and definitions before moving into more detailed discussions on common mental health disorders, therapeutic communication techniques, medication management, legal and ethical issues, and much more. Each chapter is crafted with the learner in mind, featuring real-life case studies, interactive questions, and key takeaways that reinforce learning and application in clinical settings.

Our Hope

My hope is that by the end of this book, you will not only have gained a solid foundation in mental health nursing but will also be equipped to face the challenges and rewards of this field with confidence and empathy. Whether you are a student, an educator, or a practicing nurse, "Mental Health Nursing Made Easy" is designed to be a resource you turn to time and again for guidance and inspiration.

Thank you for choosing to explore the enriching field of mental health nursing. May this book serve as your companion and guide on this important journey.

Table of Contents

Introduction

Welcome to "Mental Health Nursing Made Easy," a comprehensive guide designed to demystify the complexities of mental health nursing and make it accessible to everyone from nursing students and practicing nurses to general readers interested in mental health care. This book aims to bridge the gap between advanced theoretical knowledge and practical application in everyday clinical settings.

Mental health nursing is a vital and dynamic field, essential for the well-being of individuals and communities. As our understanding of mental health continues to evolve, so too does the role of the nurse, who often stands at the forefront of care and support for those affected by mental health issues. Whether you are starting your journey in nursing education, seeking to refine your professional practice, or simply interested in understanding more about mental health, this book is tailored for you.

In the pages that follow, you will find detailed explanations of common mental health disorders, from anxiety and depression to bipolar disorder and schizophrenia. We will explore effective communication techniques, delve into medication management, and discuss crucial legal and ethical considerations. The content is enriched with real-life case studies and practical examples that illustrate key concepts and show how they can be applied in real-world scenarios.

This book is structured to be a resource that you can turn to time and again, whether for learning new information, refreshing your knowledge, or finding guidance in your daily clinical practice. Our goal is to provide you with a solid foundation in mental health nursing, presented in a clear, concise, and engaging manner.

As we embark on this journey together, remember that the field of mental health nursing is not just about managing illness but is also deeply involved in fostering resilience, promoting wellness, and enhancing the quality of life for individuals and their families. Let's begin by laying down the basics and progressively building a comprehensive understanding that you can carry forward into your careers and daily lives.

Thank you for choosing to explore this exciting and rewarding field with us. Your commitment to learning and understanding mental health nursing can make a significant difference in many lives.

Importance of mental health nursing

Mental health nursing plays a crucial role in healthcare, providing vital support to individuals coping with mental health disorders and contributing significantly to public health. Here are some key points highlighting the importance of mental health nursing:

1. Holistic Patient Care

Mental health nurses approach patient care holistically, addressing both psychological and physical aspects of well-being. They play a pivotal role in assessing mental health needs, formulating care plans, and implementing treatments that consider the entire person, not just their symptoms. This comprehensive care supports patients' overall health and well-being, enhancing their ability to manage everyday life.

2. Early Identification and Intervention

Mental health nurses are often on the front lines, in positions to identify mental health issues early. Early detection of mental health conditions can lead to interventions that significantly alter the course of an illness, potentially reducing severity and improving quality of life. This early intervention can decrease the need for more intensive services later and can be pivotal in crisis situations.

3. Advocacy and Empowerment

Mental health nurses act as advocates for their patients, navigating complex healthcare systems and helping to secure necessary resources. They empower patients by educating them about their conditions and care options, thereby enabling informed decision-making and promoting self-care practices that support long-term health.

4. Reducing Stigma and Promoting Mental Health Awareness

Mental health nurses play a vital role in reducing stigma associated with mental illness through education and community outreach. By providing accurate information and challenging misconceptions, they foster a more understanding and supportive environment for individuals experiencing mental health issues.

5. Continuous Care and Support

Mental health nurses provide continuous, often long-term care and support for patients, helping them manage their conditions effectively over time. This includes monitoring treatment efficacy, providing therapeutic interventions, and adjusting care plans as patients' needs change. This ongoing support is essential for maintaining stability and preventing relapse.

6. Innovation and Research

Mental health nurses contribute to the advancement of mental health care through participation in research and innovation. They are involved in studies that explore new treatments, interventions, and care models, driving improvements that can lead to better patient outcomes across the healthcare system.

7. Crisis Management

In acute mental health crises, mental health nurses are essential. They provide immediate, skilled care and intervention, helping to stabilize patients who are a risk to themselves or others and ensuring they receive the appropriate level of care.

8. Community and Public Health Improvement

Mental health nurses play an integral role in public health by participating in preventative health initiatives and community programs. Their work in promoting mental health literacy and resilience helps improve community health outcomes and reduces the burden on healthcare systems.

In summary, mental health nursing is not only critical for the management and treatment of mental illnesses but also plays a broad, integrative role in improving healthcare delivery, enhancing patient outcomes, and promoting public health. Their work is essential to creating a society where mental health is understood, valued, and effectively cared for.

How to Use this book

"Mental Health Nursing Made Easy" is designed to be a user-friendly resource for individuals at different levels of their nursing career—from students just beginning their journey in mental health nursing to seasoned practitioners looking to refresh or enhance their knowledge. Here's a guide on how to get the most out of this book:

1. Read Sequentially or Selectively

- **For Beginners:** If you are new to mental health nursing, it's beneficial to read the book sequentially. Start from the first chapter and progress through to the end. This approach helps build your foundational knowledge before moving on to more complex topics.

- **For Experienced Professionals:** If you have experience in mental health nursing, you may prefer to use this book as a reference. Feel free to jump directly to specific chapters or sections that are most relevant to your current needs or interests.

2. Utilize the Case Studies and Examples

- Each chapter contains case studies and practical examples that illustrate key concepts and show how they can be applied in real-world settings. Engage with these narratives by considering the questions posed at the end of each case study, which are designed to encourage critical thinking and practical application.

3. Refer to the Glossary and Appendices

- The glossary at the end of the book provides definitions of key terms used throughout the text. If you come across unfamiliar jargon while reading, use the glossary to help understand these terms.

- Appendices include additional resources such as checklists, templates, and further readings that can enhance your learning and provide tools for your practice.

4. Interactive Learning

- Engage actively with the content. Highlight important points, make notes in the margins, and don't hesitate to write down any questions that arise as you read. This interactive approach can deepen your understanding and retention of the material.

5. Practice the Techniques

- Where practical skills and techniques are described, try them out in a simulated environment or, if possible, under supervision in your clinical practice. Hands-on practice will help you internalize the skills and gain confidence.

6. Join Discussions or Study Groups

- If you're studying as part of a course or professional group, discuss the content with peers. Sharing insights and challenges can enhance your learning experience and provide diverse perspectives on the material.

7. Stay Updated

- The field of mental health nursing is constantly evolving. Use this book as a foundation, but stay informed about new research and developments in the field through journals, online courses, and professional associations.

8. Feedback Loop

- Reflect on how the concepts learned from the book apply to your experiences in clinical settings. This reflection will help integrate theory with practice and improve your clinical judgment.

By using this book as a guide, you can enhance your understanding of mental health nursing and develop the skills necessary to deliver compassionate, effective care to those in need. Whether you're reading cover-to-cover or dipping in to tackle specific challenges in your practice, "Mental Health Nursing Made Easy" aims to be a valuable resource in your educational and professional journey.

Chapter 1: Introduction to Mental Health Nursing

What is Mental Health Nursing?

Mental health nursing, also known as psychiatric nursing, is a specialized field of nursing that involves caring for people of all ages experiencing mental illnesses or distress. These can include disorders such as schizophrenia, bipolar disorder, depression, anxiety, and others. Mental health nurses play a critical role in the healthcare team, working to support treatment plans and contribute to the well-being of patients.

Key Aspects of Mental Health Nursing Include:

1. Assessment of Mental Health Needs:

- Mental health nurses assess patients to determine their mental health status and needs. This involves evaluating psychological symptoms, personal and family history, and the social context of the patient's life.

2. Development and Implementation of Care Plans:

- Nurses collaborate with patients to develop tailored care plans. These plans often include therapeutic interventions, medication management, counseling, and other support services designed to address specific mental health needs.

3. Therapeutic Communication:

- Effective communication is crucial in mental health nursing. Nurses use a range of communication skills to build rapport, encourage patients to express their feelings, and support individuals in understanding and managing their conditions.

4. Administration of Psychiatric Medication:

- Administering medication and monitoring its effects is a fundamental part of the role. Mental health nurses must understand pharmacology and its application in treating psychiatric disorders to manage side effects and ensure compliance with treatment regimens.

5. Advocacy:

- Mental health nurses advocate for the rights and needs of their patients. This can include ensuring that patients have access to necessary healthcare services, supporting them in voicing their concerns, and educating them and their families about mental health conditions and their rights within the healthcare system.

6. Crisis Intervention:

- Nurses often manage crises, which can involve acute behavioral disturbances or suicidal ideation. They are trained to de-escalate crises safely and effectively, often coordinating care with other professionals to provide comprehensive crisis intervention services.

7. Education and Health Promotion:

- Mental health nurses also focus on educating patients, families, and communities about mental health conditions to promote health, reduce stigma, and prevent illness. They provide tools and strategies to improve mental health through lifestyle changes, stress management techniques, and healthy coping mechanisms.

8. Multi-disciplinary Team Collaboration:

- They work collaboratively with a multidisciplinary team that can include psychiatrists, psychologists, social workers, and occupational therapists to provide holistic care.

9. Continuous Care and Rehabilitation:

- Focused on supporting patients' long-term wellness, mental health nurses help develop rehabilitation goals that foster recovery, community integration, and improved quality of life.

Mental health nursing requires a compassionate approach, resilience, and a deep understanding of human behavior and psychology. Nurses in this field are often celebrated for their empathy, patience, and ability to connect with people undergoing significant distress, helping them navigate the path towards recovery and maintaining long-term mental health.

History and evolution of the field

The history and evolution of mental health nursing reflect broader changes in society's understanding of mental health and the treatments deemed appropriate and humane. This evolution has seen a shift from punitive and often cruel treatments to a more compassionate, therapeutic approach that recognizes the dignity and potential for recovery of individuals with mental illnesses.

Early History

- **Ancient Times to 18th Century:** Historically, mental illness was often misunderstood, with sufferers subjected to superstition and fear. Treatments varied from the brutal (such as exorcisms or confinement) to the bizarre, based on the balance of bodily humors, astrological factors, and spiritual explanations.

- **19th Century:** The 1800s marked a significant shift towards more humane treatment of the mentally ill, largely due to reformers like Philippe Pinel in France and Dorothea Dix in the United States. They advocated for better conditions in asylums and more compassionate care. This period saw the construction of many new psychiatric institutions where the care focus was custodial rather than therapeutic.

Transition to a More Modern Approach

- **Early 20th Century:** Advances in medicine and psychology, including the development of Freudian psychoanalysis, began influencing mental health care. However, treatments like electroconvulsive therapy (ECT) and lobotomies were also developed during this time, reflecting an ongoing exploration of more radical approaches to mental health problems.

- **Mid-20th Century:** The introduction of the first antipsychotic medications in the 1950s, such as chlorpromazine, revolutionized mental health care. These medications allowed many patients to manage symptoms effectively enough to live outside hospital settings. This period also saw the growth of the community mental health movement, especially following the deinstitutionalization policies in the 1960s and 70s in the United States, which aimed to integrate people with mental health conditions into the community and close large psychiatric hospitals.

Evolution of Mental Health Nursing

- **Early Roles:** Initially, nurses in mental health settings acted primarily as custodians and caretakers, with little formal training in therapeutic techniques or psychiatric theory.

- **Professional Development:** Over time, as understanding of mental health advanced, so did the role of the mental health nurse. Formal training programs and certification processes were established. The role expanded from custodial care to include therapeutic and psychiatric care, emphasizing patient rights, informed consent, and ethical considerations.

- **Therapeutic and Holistic Approaches:** From the late 20th century to today, mental health nursing has increasingly embraced a holistic and patient-centered approach. This includes the use of therapeutic communication, psychoeducation, psychosocial interventions, and an emphasis on recovery-oriented care.

- **Advanced Practice:** Today, advanced practice psychiatric nurses can perform a wide range of functions, including diagnosis and treatment of mental illnesses, conducting psychotherapy, and prescribing medications.

Current Trends

Today, mental health nursing is a vital and dynamic field that combines a range of therapeutic, pharmacological, and interpersonal interventions to provide comprehensive care. The focus is increasingly on evidence-based practices, cultural sensitivity, and the integration of technology and digital health tools into care delivery. Nurses work in diverse settings, from hospitals and community clinics to private practices and telehealth, reflecting the broad scope and adaptability of the field.

The ongoing development of mental health nursing continues to be influenced by changes in healthcare policy, societal attitudes towards mental health, and advancements in medical research, ensuring that the field adapts to meet the evolving needs of society.

Key principles and goals of mental health nursing

Mental health nursing is built upon several foundational principles and goals that guide the practice and ensure that it delivers compassionate, effective, and ethical care. These principles and goals help mental health nurses in making clinical decisions and shaping the care they provide to meet the diverse needs of individuals with mental health conditions.

Key Principles of Mental Health Nursing

1. **Holistic Care**: Mental health nursing recognizes the importance of addressing the whole person, considering their physical, emotional, psychological, social, and spiritual needs. This approach acknowledges the complex interplay between various aspects of an individual's life and health.

2. **Empathy and Compassion**: Nurses must approach each patient with empathy and compassion, striving to understand the patient's experiences and feelings without judgment. This helps build a therapeutic alliance that can significantly improve care outcomes.

3. **Patient-Centered Care**: This principle involves tailoring the healthcare process to fit individual patient's preferences, needs, and values, and ensuring that patient values guide all clinical decisions. This often includes involving patients in their care planning and decision-making processes.

4. **Respect for Dignity**: Every individual, regardless of their mental health condition, has the right to be treated with dignity and respect. This includes respecting their privacy, confidentiality, and personal choices.

5. **Advocacy**: Nurses often advocate for the rights and needs of their patients, especially in situations where patients might not be able to speak for themselves. This can involve advocating for access to necessary healthcare services or supporting patients' rights within the healthcare system.

6. **Safety**: Ensuring the safety of patients is paramount in mental health nursing. This includes managing risks associated with mental health conditions, safeguarding against self-harm or harm to others, and creating a safe therapeutic environment.

7. **Evidence-Based Practice**: Mental health nursing relies on current research and best practices to guide interventions and treatments. This ensures that the care provided is based on the latest and most effective approaches.

Goals of Mental Health Nursing

1. **Promotion of Mental Health**: Nurses work not only to treat mental illness but also to promote mental health and well-being through education, early intervention, and the encouragement of healthy lifestyle choices.

2. **Prevention of Mental Health Problems**: This includes implementing strategies to reduce the incidence of mental health conditions and addressing risk factors that might lead to such conditions.

3. **Recovery-Oriented Care**: A major goal is to support the recovery of individuals, which involves empowering them to regain control over their lives and achieve their personal goals in the context of the recovery from mental illness.

4. **Symptom Management**: Mental health nurses help patients manage the symptoms of their mental illness, which can include administering medication, providing psychotherapy, and teaching coping strategies.

5. **Improving Quality of Life**: Beyond managing symptoms, mental health nursing aims to enhance the overall quality of life for individuals, helping them to integrate or reintegrate into society, maintain relationships, and pursue meaningful activities.

6. **Education**: Educating patients, families, and the broader community about mental health is a crucial goal. This education can demystify mental health conditions, reduce stigma, and promote a more informed and supportive community environment.

By adhering to these principles and striving to meet these goals, mental health nurses play a critical role in the healthcare system, contributing significantly to the well-being of individuals with mental health challenges.

Chapter 2: Understanding Common Mental Health Disorders

Anxiety Disorders

Anxiety disorders are among the most common mental health conditions and can significantly impact a person's daily functioning and quality of life. Understanding the different types of anxiety disorders, their symptoms, and effective nursing interventions is crucial in providing appropriate care and support.

Types of Anxiety Disorders

1. **Generalized Anxiety Disorder (GAD)**: Characterized by chronic, excessive worry about a variety of topics, events, or activities. Worry is often disproportionate to the actual likelihood or impact of the feared events.

2. **Panic Disorder**: Involves recurrent, unexpected panic attacks—sudden surges of overwhelming fear and physical symptoms, such as heart palpitations, chest pain, dizziness, or abdominal distress.

3. **Phobias**: Involves intense fear or aversion to specific objects or situations. Common phobias include fear of heights, spiders, flying, and crowded spaces.

4. **Social Anxiety Disorder (Social Phobia)**: A significant fear of social or performance situations, where embarrassment may occur.

5. **Obsessive-Compulsive Disorder (OCD)**: Although categorized separately in the DSM-5, OCD is often discussed with anxiety disorders. It features uncontrollable, recurring thoughts (obsessions) and behaviors (compulsions) that the person feels the urge to repeat over and over.

6. **Post-Traumatic Stress Disorder (PTSD)**: Can develop after exposure to a traumatic event, with symptoms including flashbacks, severe anxiety, and uncontrollable thoughts about the event.

Symptoms of Anxiety Disorders

- Excessive worrying or fear
- Feeling agitated or restless
- Fatigue
- Difficulty concentrating
- Irritability
- Tense muscles
- Trouble sleeping
- Panic attacks
- Avoidance of certain situations or activities

Nursing Interventions for Anxiety Disorders

Assessment and Monitoring:

- Conduct thorough assessments to identify symptoms, triggers, and the impact on daily functioning.

- Regularly monitor the patient's mental status and response to treatments.

Psychoeducation:

- Educate patients and families about anxiety disorders, treatment options, and coping strategies.

- Discuss the role of medications, therapy, and lifestyle changes in managing anxiety.

Therapeutic Communication:

- Use a calm, reassuring approach to help reduce anxiety symptoms.

- Encourage patients to express their feelings and concerns, which can alleviate anxiety.

Behavioral Interventions:

- Teach relaxation techniques such as deep breathing, progressive muscle relaxation, and mindfulness meditation.

- Encourage gradual exposure to feared objects or situations, if applicable, under controlled conditions.

Medication Management:

- Assist in the administration of anti-anxiety medications as prescribed and monitor for side effects.

- Educate patients about the importance of adherence to prescribed treatments and the potential impact of medications.

Supportive Care:

- Provide a supportive and safe environment. Reduce stressors that may trigger anxiety symptoms.

- Offer support through psychotherapy sessions or support groups where patients can learn from others facing similar challenges.

Referral:

- Refer patients to mental health specialists such as psychiatrists, psychologists, or therapists for further evaluation and treatment.

- Connect patients with community resources to support their recovery and improve their quality of life.

By implementing these interventions, mental health nurses can effectively support individuals with anxiety disorders, helping them to manage their symptoms and improve their overall mental health and well-being.

Depression

Depression is a common and serious mental health condition that negatively affects how a person feels, thinks, and handles daily activities. It is crucial for mental health nurses to be proficient in identifying and managing depression in clinical settings to help patients navigate their recovery effectively.

Identifying Depression

Symptoms of Depression may include, but are not limited to:

- Persistent sad, anxious, or "empty" mood
- Feelings of hopelessness or pessimism
- Irritability
- Feelings of guilt, worthlessness, or helplessness
- Loss of interest or pleasure in hobbies and activities
- Decreased energy or fatigue
- Moving or talking more slowly
- Difficulty concentrating, remembering, or making decisions
- Sleep disturbances (insomnia, early-morning wakefulness, or oversleeping)
- Appetite and/or weight changes
- Thoughts of death or suicide, or suicide attempts

- Aches or pains, headaches, cramps, or digestive problems without a clear physical cause and/or that do not ease even with treatment

Diagnosis is typically made based on the patient's history and clinical presentation. Standardized screening tools like the Patient Health Questionnaire (PHQ-9) can be employed to assess the severity of depression.

Managing Depression in Clinical Settings

Assessment and Monitoring:

- Conduct a comprehensive assessment to confirm the diagnosis, identify the severity of the symptoms, and plan appropriate interventions.

- Regularly monitor the patient's mood, behavior, and response to treatment.

Psychoeducation:

- Educate the patient and their family about depression, including its symptoms, causes, and treatments.

- Discuss the role of various treatment modalities and the importance of adhering to prescribed therapies.

Medication Management:

- Antidepressants may be prescribed by physicians or psychiatrists. Nurses play a critical role in managing these medications, monitoring for side effects, and evaluating the effectiveness of treatment.

- Educate patients about the potential side effects and the expected timeline for improvement, as antidepressants typically take several weeks to show benefits.

Therapeutic Communication:

- Employ empathetic listening to provide emotional support.

- Encourage patients to express their feelings and thoughts, which can be therapeutic in itself.

Behavioral Therapies:

- Cognitive Behavioral Therapy (CBT), which involves working to change negative patterns of thinking and behavior, is often effective.

- Interpersonal Therapy (IPT) focuses on improving troubled personal relationships that may be contributing to or exacerbating the depression.

Lifestyle Modifications:

- Encourage regular physical activity, which has been shown to have antidepressant effects.

- Support the development of a structured daily routine including sufficient sleep, balanced nutrition, and social interaction.

Suicide Risk Assessment:

- Always assess for the risk of self-harm or suicide, particularly in patients showing severe symptoms of depression or those expressing thoughts of death.

- Develop a safety plan that includes removing means for self-harm and providing emergency contacts.

Referral and Coordination of Care:

- Collaborate with psychiatrists, psychologists, and other healthcare providers to ensure a multidisciplinary approach to treatment.

- Refer patients to mental health specialists when more specialized or intensive care is needed.

Support Systems:

- Connect patients with community resources such as support groups or community-based services.

- Encourage participation in activities that connect them with others, reducing isolation and improving mood.

By integrating these strategies, mental health nurses can provide effective care and support for patients experiencing depression, enhancing their potential for recovery and the quality of their life.

Bipolar Disorder

Bipolar disorder is a complex mental health condition characterized by significant mood swings that include emotional highs (mania or hypomania) and lows (depression). These mood swings can affect sleep, energy levels, behavior, judgment, and the ability to think clearly. Episodes of mood swings may occur rarely or multiple times a year. While most individuals will experience some emotional symptoms between episodes, some may not experience any.

Overview of Bipolar Disorder

Types of Bipolar Disorder:

1. **Bipolar I Disorder:** This type is characterized by manic episodes lasting at least 7 days or by manic symptoms that are so severe immediate hospital care is needed. Usually, depressive episodes occur as well, typically lasting at least 2 weeks.

2. **Bipolar II Disorder:** A pattern of depressive episodes and hypomanic episodes, but not the full-blown manic episodes that are typical of Bipolar I Disorder.

3. **Cyclothymic Disorder (Cyclothymia):** Periods of hypomanic symptoms as well as periods of depressive symptoms lasting for at least 2 years (1 year in children and adolescents); however, the symptoms do not meet the diagnostic requirements for a hypomanic episode and a depressive episode.

Common Symptoms:

- **Manic phase symptoms:** Increased energy, euphoria, decreased need for sleep, grandiosity, increased talkativeness, racing thoughts, distractibility, aggressive behavior, agitation, or impulsivity.

- **Depressive phase symptoms:** Low energy and motivation, feelings of sadness or emptiness, insomnia or excessive sleeping, irritability, chronic pain without a known cause, loss of interest in activities once enjoyed, feelings of worthlessness or guilt.

Treatment Strategies for Bipolar Disorder

Medication Management:

- **Mood Stabilizers:** Typically the first line of treatment; includes medications such as lithium and valproate.

- **Antipsychotics:** If symptoms of mania or depression persist despite treatment with other medications, antipsychotics may be effective.

- **Antidepressants:** Used cautiously in bipolar disorder management due to the risk of triggering a manic episode. Often prescribed in combination with a mood stabilizer.

- **Benzodiazepines:** May be used to calm or sedate an individual during manic episodes on a short-term basis.

Psychotherapy:

- **Cognitive Behavioral Therapy (CBT):** Helps individuals in identifying and changing harmful or negative thought patterns and behaviors.

- **Psychoeducation:** Patients and families learn about bipolar disorder and its management, which can help reduce problems and improve adherence to treatment plans.

- **Family Therapy:** Helps family members understand the disorder and provides strategies to support their loved one.

- **Interpersonal and Social Rhythm Therapy (IPSRT):** Focuses on stabilizing daily rhythms such as sleeping, eating, and activity schedules, which can help manage the mood swings.

Lifestyle Modifications and Self-Management:

- **Routine Management:** Encourage patients to keep a consistent routine, including sleep schedules.

- **Exercise:** Regular physical activity can help manage symptoms of depression, reduce stress, and improve overall health.

- **Monitoring Mood Swings:** Use of mood diaries to track moods, triggers, and responses to treatments.

- **Avoiding Triggers:** Minimize high-stress situations, maintain good sleep hygiene, and avoid stimulants like caffeine.

Hospitalization:

- May be necessary during severe manic or depressive episodes if a person is behaving dangerously, has thoughts of suicide, or becomes detached from reality (psychotic).

Continued Support and Monitoring:

- Regular follow-ups with mental health professionals to monitor symptoms and make necessary adjustments to the treatment plan.

- Participation in support groups or community services can provide additional emotional support and education.

Bipolar disorder requires a comprehensive treatment plan tailored to the individual's needs. This often involves a combination of medication, psychotherapy, lifestyle changes, and possibly hospitalization to manage symptoms effectively and improve quality of life.

Schizophrenia

Schizophrenia is a serious mental disorder that affects how a person thinks, feels, and behaves. People with schizophrenia may seem like they have lost touch with reality, which can be distressing for them and for their family and friends. The disorder is complex, involving a range of cognitive, behavioral, and emotional dysfunctions, and it requires careful and comprehensive management.

Understanding Schizophrenia

Symptoms of Schizophrenia can be divided into three broad categories:

- **Positive Symptoms**: These include hallucinations (such as hearing voices), delusions (false beliefs), thought disorders (unusual or dysfunctional ways of thinking), and movement disorders (agitated body movements).

- **Negative Symptoms**: These refer to reductions or deficits in normal emotional and behavioral states, such as reduced speaking even when required to interact, lack of emotional expression, diminished ability to initiate and sustain planned activities, and social withdrawal.

- **Cognitive Symptoms**: These involve problems with attention, certain types of memory, and the executive functions that allow us to plan and organize. Cognitive impairment can significantly affect a person's ability to function and is one of the most disabling aspects of the disease.

Causes of Schizophrenia include a combination of genetic, brain chemistry, and environmental factors. These factors contribute to a dysfunction in the neural circuits that manage sensory processing, emotions, and social behavior.

Effective Nursing Care for Schizophrenia

Assessment and Monitoring:

- Conduct comprehensive assessments to identify the specific symptoms and needs of each patient.

Regular monitoring is essential to evaluate the effectiveness of treatments and any changes in symptoms.

- Use of standardized assessment tools can help in documenting symptom severity and response to treatment.

Medication Management:

- Antipsychotic medications are the cornerstone of schizophrenia treatment and are effective in reducing or eliminating positive symptoms. Nurses play a key role in administering these medications, monitoring their side effects, and educating patients about the importance of adhering to prescribed treatment.

- Regular assessment for side effects, particularly extrapyramidal symptoms (like tremors or rigidity), metabolic issues, and cardiovascular health is crucial.

Psychoeducation:

- Educating patients and families about schizophrenia and its management can empower them and improve treatment outcomes. Understanding the disease helps reduce stigma and can motivate adherence to treatment plans.

Therapeutic Communication:

- Establishing a trusting relationship through consistent, supportive interactions can help manage the symptoms of schizophrenia. Effective communication also involves being patient and clear, using simple and direct language, and listening actively.

Supportive Therapies:

- Cognitive Behavioral Therapy (CBT) can help patients manage the symptoms of schizophrenia by teaching them to recognize and change distorted thoughts and behaviors.

- Social skills training may be part of the therapeutic approach to help patients improve their communication and interpersonal skills.

Management of Daily Living:

- Nurses can assist patients with schizophrenia in developing skills for daily living, such as personal hygiene, cooking, and managing finances, which are often impaired by the cognitive symptoms of schizophrenia.

Crisis Intervention:

- Be prepared to respond to acute episodes or crises, which might include severe psychotic symptoms or potential harm to the patient or others. Ensuring safety and providing immediate care in such instances are vital roles of the nursing staff.

Long-term Support and Rehabilitation:

- Focus on rehabilitation strategies that help reintegrate patients into the community, such as vocational training and job placement services.

- Encourage participation in community activities and social groups to enhance social support networks.

Lifestyle and Well-being:

- Encouraging healthy lifestyles, including regular physical activity, balanced nutrition, and adequate sleep, can help manage symptoms and improve overall well-being.

- Monitor and support efforts to reduce or eliminate substance use, as alcohol and drugs can exacerbate symptoms or interfere with medications.

Effective nursing care for schizophrenia involves a multifaceted approach, combining medication management, patient and family education, supportive therapies, and practical assistance with everyday activities. By addressing both the medical and psychosocial needs of patients, mental health nurses play a crucial role in helping individuals with schizophrenia lead more stable and satisfying lives.

Post-Traumatic Stress Disorder (PTSD)

Post-Traumatic Stress Disorder (PTSD) is a mental health condition triggered by experiencing or witnessing a terrifying event. Symptoms may include flashbacks, nightmares, severe anxiety, as well as uncontrollable thoughts about the event. Managing PTSD effectively requires a comprehensive approach that includes identifying symptoms, applying appropriate clinical management strategies, and implementing targeted nursing interventions.

Symptoms of PTSD

PTSD symptoms are generally grouped into four types:

1. **Intrusion Symptoms:**

   - Recurrent, involuntary, and intrusive distressing memories of the traumatic event.

   - Repeated distressing dreams related to the content or emotions of the traumatic event.

   - Flashbacks or other dissociative reactions in which the individual feels or acts as if the traumatic event were recurring.

2. **Avoidance Symptoms:**

   - Efforts to avoid distressing memories, thoughts, or feelings about or closely associated with the traumatic event.

   - Efforts to avoid external reminders (people, places, conversations, activities, objects, situations) that arouse distressing memories, thoughts, or feelings about or closely associated with the traumatic event.

3. **Negative Changes in Cognition and Mood:**

- Inability to remember an important aspect of the traumatic event (typically due to dissociative amnesia and not to other factors such as head injury, alcohol, or drugs).

- Persistent and exaggerated negative beliefs or expectations about oneself, others, or the world.

- Persistent, distorted cognitions about the cause or consequences of the traumatic event that lead the individual to blame themselves or others.

- Persistent negative emotional state (e.g., fear, horror, anger, guilt, or shame).

- Markedly diminished interest or participation in significant activities.

- Feelings of detachment or estrangement from others.

- Persistent inability to experience positive emotions.

4. **Alterations in Arousal and Reactivity:**

- Irritable behavior and angry outbursts (with little or no provocation) typically expressed as verbal or physical aggression toward people or objects.

- Reckless or self-destructive behavior.

- Hypervigilance.

- Exaggerated startle response.

- Problems with concentration.

- Sleep disturbance (e.g., difficulty falling or staying asleep or restless sleep).

Identifying and Managing PTSD in Clinical Settings

Clinical Management:

- **Assessment Tools:** Use structured interviews and validated assessment tools such as the PTSD Checklist (PCL) or the Clinician-Administered PTSD Scale (CAPS) to diagnose PTSD and monitor treatment progress.

- **Psychoeducation:** Educate the patient and their family about PTSD symptoms and treatment options, which can demystify the condition and reduce feelings of guilt or blame.

- **Medication:** Consider the use of medications like SSRIs (selective serotonin reuptake inhibitors) or SNRIs (serotonin-norepinephrine reuptake inhibitors) to manage symptoms.

- **Psychotherapy:** Techniques such as Cognitive Behavioral Therapy (CBT), Eye Movement Desensitization and Reprocessing (EMDR), and Prolonged Exposure Therapy have been proven effective in treating PTSD.

Nursing Interventions for PTSD

Supportive Care:

- **Establish Safety:** Create a safe and predictable environment that can help reduce symptoms of hypervigilance and anxiety.

- **Active Listening:** Provide a supportive presence that encourages patients to talk about their trauma at their own pace and comfort level.

- **Trauma-Informed Care:** Be aware of and sensitive to trauma-related issues present in PTSD patients. Avoid actions that could re-traumatize the patient.

Behavioral Strategies:

- **Relaxation Techniques:** Teach and practice techniques such as deep breathing, progressive muscle relaxation, and mindfulness to help manage anxiety and stress.

- **Sleep Hygiene:** Assist in developing routines that promote healthy sleep, given that sleep disturbances are a common symptom of PTSD.

Advocacy:

- **Coordinate Care:** Work closely with psychiatrists, psychologists, and social workers to ensure a comprehensive, multi-disciplinary approach to care.

- **Community Resources:** Help connect patients with community resources and PTSD support groups, which can provide additional layers of support.

Monitoring and Follow-Up:

- **Regular Monitoring:** Keep track of the patient's symptoms and treatment responses. Adjust care plans based on progress or any setbacks.

- **Education on Coping Strategies:** Continuously educate patients on coping mechanisms and how to apply them in everyday life to manage symptoms effectively.

Nursing care for PTSD is complex and multifaceted, requiring empathy, patience, and a well-coordinated approach among healthcare providers to help patients recover and regain control over their lives.

Obsessive-Compulsive Disorder (OCD)

Obsessive-Compulsive Disorder (OCD) is a chronic mental health condition characterized by uncontrollable, recurring thoughts (obsessions) and behaviors (compulsions) that the sufferer feels compelled to repeat over and over. These symptoms can significantly disrupt daily activities and cause considerable distress.

Symptoms of OCD

Obsessions are intrusive and unwanted thoughts, images, or urges that cause significant anxiety or distress. Common obsessions include fears of contamination, aggressive or horrific thoughts about harming oneself or others, and desires for orderliness and symmetry.

Compulsions are repetitive behaviors or mental acts that a person feels driven to perform in response to an obsession, according to rules that must be applied rigidly.

These behaviors often include washing and cleaning, counting, checking, demanding reassurances, or performing the same action repeatedly. The purpose of these behaviors is to reduce distress related to obsessions or prevent some dreaded event or situation; however, these behaviors are not connected in a realistic way with the issue they are intended to address or are clearly excessive.

Identifying and Managing OCD in Clinical Settings

Assessment Tools:

- Use standardized assessment tools such as the Yale-Brown Obsessive Compulsive Scale (Y-BOCS) to evaluate the severity of OCD and monitor treatment outcomes.

Psychoeducation:

- Educate patients and their families about OCD, its nature, the role of obsessions and compulsions, and treatment options. Understanding the disorder can reduce feelings of shame or isolation and increase treatment adherence.

Medication Management:

- SSRIs (Selective Serotonin Reuptake Inhibitors) are commonly used to help reduce the symptoms of OCD. Other medications like clomipramine, a tricyclic antidepressant, may also be considered for more severe cases.

- Monitor the effectiveness of medication therapy and manage side effects, which are crucial roles for nurses.

Cognitive-Behavioral Therapy (CBT):

- CBT, particularly Exposure and Response Prevention (ERP), is highly effective for treating OCD. ERP involves exposing the patient to the source of their anxiety (the obsessions) without allowing them to engage in the compulsive behavior usually performed to reduce the anxiety.

Nursing Interventions for OCD

Supportive Care:

- **Active Listening:** Offer a nonjudgmental, supportive presence that encourages patients to express their thoughts and feelings about their obsessions and compulsions.

- **Validation of Feelings:** Validate the patient's experiences and feelings while helping them understand that their compulsions are a symptom of their disorder.

Behavioral Strategies:

- **Routine Management:** Assist in developing structured daily routines that help reduce the opportunity for compulsive behaviors. Regular routines can provide a sense of control and reduce anxiety levels.

- **Stress Management:** Introduce and practice stress-reduction techniques, such as mindfulness and relaxation exercises, to help manage the anxiety that fuels obsessions and compulsions.

Patient Education:

- **Skill Development:** Teach skills to resist compulsions and manage obsessive thoughts independently, emphasizing the importance of gradual progress and the application of CBT techniques.

- **Health Education:** Provide comprehensive education on the importance of maintaining a balanced lifestyle, including proper diet, exercise, and sleep, which can positively impact overall mental health.

Monitoring and Follow-Up:

- **Ongoing Assessment:** Regularly assess the patient's mental state and symptom severity to gauge treatment progress and adjust care plans accordingly.

- **Support System Building:** Encourage engagement with support groups or connect patients with community resources to enhance support outside the clinical setting.

Crisis Management:

- Be prepared to intervene if the patient experiences intense distress or if symptoms significantly interfere with their daily life, including ensuring safety and providing immediate emotional and therapeutic support.

In managing OCD, the integration of medication, behavioral therapies, patient education, and supportive nursing care can significantly enhance treatment outcomes. Nurses play a critical role in managing daily care, providing emotional support, and educating patients on how to cope with and manage OCD effectively.

Chapter 3: Therapeutic Communication Techniques

Basics of effective communication in mental health nursing

Effective communication is essential in mental health nursing, as it forms the foundation of therapeutic relationships and ensures that care is patient-centered and respectful. It involves more than just talking; it includes listening, observing, empathizing, and engaging in a way that promotes understanding and trust. Here are the basics of effective communication tailored for mental health nursing:

1. Active Listening

Active listening means paying full attention to the patient, not only to the words but also to the tone of voice and body language. It involves listening without judgment and acknowledging the patient's feelings and thoughts. This can help the patient feel valued and understood, which is crucial for building trust.

2. Empathy

Empathy involves understanding and sharing the feelings of another person. In mental health nursing, showing empathy means acknowledging the patient's emotional state and demonstrating understanding and concern. This reassures patients that their feelings are valid and that they are in a safe space to share their thoughts.

3. Clarity and Simplicity

Communicating in clear, simple language is important, especially when discussing complex issues like treatment plans or diagnoses. Avoid medical jargon unless you are sure the patient understands, and even then, it's often better to use layman's terms. Be concise and direct, and always check for understanding.

4. Nonverbal Communication

Nonverbal cues, including facial expressions, body posture, and eye contact, play a significant role in communication. Positive nonverbal communication can make the therapeutic interaction more engaging and comforting. For example, maintaining a relaxed posture and appropriate eye contact conveys openness and attentiveness.

5. Patience

Patients with mental health issues might have difficulty expressing themselves, may speak more slowly, or have trouble finding the right words. Showing patience by giving them time to articulate their thoughts without rushing them is key in facilitating effective communication.

6. Respect and Dignity

Always address patients by their preferred name or title unless invited to do otherwise. Respect their views, even if they differ from your own, and avoid making assumptions based on stereotypes or diagnoses. Respecting a patient's autonomy and opinions fosters a more productive therapeutic relationship.

7. Asking Questions

Use open-ended questions that require more than a yes or no response to encourage patients to elaborate on their feelings and experiences. This technique can help uncover additional information that might be crucial for their care.

8. Therapeutic Silence

Silence can be a powerful tool in mental health communication. It gives patients time to think and gather their thoughts, which can be particularly helpful when they are trying to articulate difficult emotions or memories.

9. Feedback

Offering feedback lets patients know that their communication is effective and valued. It also helps clarify that what you have understood is indeed what they intended to communicate.

10. Cultural Sensitivity

Being aware of and sensitive to the cultural backgrounds of patients is crucial. This includes understanding cultural specifics about eye contact, touch, and the patient's expectations of healthcare providers. Adapt your communication style to meet the cultural and individual needs of each patient.

Implementing these effective communication techniques in mental health nursing not only improves the quality of care but also enhances patient satisfaction, engagement in treatment, and overall outcomes. It builds a foundation of trust and respect, which are crucial for any therapeutic relationship.

Specific techniques for different mental health conditions

Effective communication techniques can vary significantly depending on the mental health condition being addressed. Tailoring communication strategies to meet the specific needs and symptoms of each condition can enhance therapeutic interactions and improve patient outcomes. Here's a look at some specific communication techniques for various mental health conditions:

1. Depression

- **Empathic Listening**: Show genuine empathy and interest in what the person is sharing, acknowledging their feelings and struggles.

- **Encouragement**: Often, individuals with depression may feel hopeless; encourage them by highlighting small achievements and strengths.

- **Simple and Clear Language**: Use clear and straightforward language to avoid adding confusion to their possibly impaired concentration and decision-making abilities.

2. Anxiety Disorders

- **Reassurance**: Provide calm and reassuring responses that help to reduce immediate anxiety and stress.

- **Grounding Techniques**: Teach and use grounding techniques during conversations to help manage acute anxiety symptoms.

- **Guided Discovery**: Use questions to help patients explore the reality of their fears and anxiety, challenging distorted perceptions and thoughts.

3. Bipolar Disorder

- **Mood Congruent Communication**: Adjust the pace and tone of conversations according to the patient's mood state (e.g., more subdued during manic phases, more energetic during depressive phases).

- **Consistency**: Maintain a consistent approach and message, helping to provide a sense of stability.

- **Clear and Structured Communication**: Especially important during manic episodes, where thought processes may be disorganized.

4. Schizophrenia

- **Simple and Direct Language**: Use straightforward language as patients may have impaired thought processes.

- **Validating Reality**: Acknowledge the patient's experiences, but gently reinforce reality to help orient them.

- **Therapeutic Silence**: Sometimes, allowing for pauses in the conversation can help patients better process their thoughts and feelings.

5. Obsessive-Compulsive Disorder (OCD)

- **Reassurance Without Enabling**: Reassure the patient of their safety and well-being without reinforcing their compulsive behaviors.

- **Encourage Open Dialogue**: Encourage them to talk about their thoughts and compulsions, which can reduce the power of these thoughts over time.

- **Patient-Centered Questioning**: Help them explore the rationale behind their behaviors and fears through careful questioning.

6. Post-Traumatic Stress Disorder (PTSD)

- **Trauma-Informed Care**: Always approach conversations with an understanding of trauma's impact and avoid any triggers.

- **Supportive Listening**: Provide a safe space for them to share their experiences at their own pace without pressure.

- **Empowerment**: Focus conversations on their strengths and ways to regain control over their lives.

7. Personality Disorders

- **Consistent Boundaries**: Clearly communicate boundaries consistently, as patients with personality disorders may test limits.

- **Reflective Listening**: Reflect emotions and thoughts expressed to show understanding and validation.

- **Managing Transference**: Be vigilant about transference and countertransference issues that can significantly impact therapeutic relationships.

These techniques should be adapted based on the patient's current state, history, and specific needs. Mental health nurses must continuously assess and adjust their communication strategies to provide the most effective and compassionate care possible. By employing condition-specific communication techniques, healthcare providers can better connect with patients, aiding significantly in their treatment and recovery process.

Role-playing scenarios to practice communication skills

Role-playing is an effective method for practicing and refining communication skills, particularly in the field of mental health nursing. It allows nurses to simulate real-life interactions with patients, providing an opportunity to apply theoretical knowledge in a controlled environment. Here are some role-playing scenarios that can help mental health nurses enhance their communication skills:

Scenario 1: Dealing with Anxiety

Situation: You are a nurse working in a mental health clinic. A patient comes in for an appointment, visibly anxious and having trouble sitting still. **Objectives**:

- Use calming communication techniques.

- Employ grounding techniques to help manage the patient's anxiety.

- Reassure the patient and provide a sense of safety.

Role Play:

- **Nurse:** "I see that you seem a bit uneasy today. Can we try a breathing exercise together to help you feel more relaxed?"

- **Patient:** "I can't calm down. It feels like my heart is racing."

- **Nurse:** "That sounds really uncomfortable. Let's breathe together. Inhale slowly... Now exhale. Let's repeat this a few times."

Scenario 2: Supporting a Patient with Depression

Situation: A patient with depression expresses feelings of hopelessness and questions the point of continuing treatment. **Objectives:**

- Show empathy and understanding.

- Motivate the patient by discussing past improvements and setting small, achievable goals.

- Encourage the patient to express their feelings and thoughts openly.

Role Play:

- **Nurse:** "It sounds like things have been really tough for you lately. What do you feel has changed since starting treatment?"

- **Patient**: "Nothing really matters; it's all pointless."

- **Nurse**: "I hear you saying that it feels pointless, and that must be really hard. Let's talk about some moments when you did feel a bit better. Sometimes, noticing small changes can help us see some light in the dark."

Scenario 3: Managing Manic Behavior in Bipolar Disorder

Situation: A patient with bipolar disorder is experiencing a manic episode, talking rapidly about many grand plans and ideas. **Objectives**:

- Use techniques to gently slow down the conversation and focus the patient.

- Maintain a calm and steady demeanor.

- Guide the patient to discuss one idea at a time.

Role Play:

- **Nurse**: "You have a lot of exciting ideas! Let's take a moment to focus on one at a time. Tell me more about your plan for starting a business."

- **Patient**: "It's going to be huge, you know, I thought about this last night and I can make millions. I just need to get some things sorted out..."

- **Nurse**: "It sounds like you've put a lot of thought into this. Let's outline some steps together that you think are necessary to get started. We can discuss each step one by one."

Scenario 4: Educating a Patient about Medication

Situation: You need to explain the importance of medication adherence to a schizophrenic patient who has been non-compliant. **Objectives**:

- Clearly explain the benefits and side effects of the medication.

- Understand and address the patient's concerns about medication.

- Encourage questions and provide reassurance.

Role Play:

- **Nurse**: "I noticed you've been hesitant about taking your medication regularly. Can you share your concerns with me?"

- **Patient**: "I don't like how they make me feel. I feel numb and not myself."

- **Nurse**: "It's important to feel like yourself, and your feelings about the medication are valid. Let's discuss how it helps with your symptoms, and maybe we can talk to your doctor about adjusting the dosage or trying a different type that might have fewer side effects."

These role-playing scenarios can help mental health nurses develop a repertoire of responses and strategies for effectively communicating with patients across a range of situations. Practicing these scenarios can build confidence, empathy, and skill in handling complex patient interactions.

Chapter 4: Medication Management

Common medications used in mental health treatment

Medication is a cornerstone of treatment for many mental health disorders, often used in conjunction with psychotherapy and other therapeutic interventions. Below is an overview of common classes of medications used in mental health treatment, along with examples of each and their general uses.

1. Antidepressants

Antidepressants are commonly used to treat depression, anxiety disorders, and other mood disorders. They generally work by altering the levels of neurotransmitters in the brain, such as serotonin, norepinephrine, and dopamine.

- **Selective Serotonin Reuptake Inhibitors (SSRIs):** e.g., Fluoxetine (Prozac), Sertraline (Zoloft), Citalopram (Celexa)

- **Serotonin and Norepinephrine Reuptake Inhibitors (SNRIs):** e.g., Venlafaxine (Effexor), Duloxetine (Cymbalta)

- **Tricyclic Antidepressants (TCAs):** e.g., Amitriptyline, Nortriptyline (Pamelor)

- **Monoamine Oxidase Inhibitors (MAOIs):** e.g., Phenelzine (Nardil), Tranylcypromine (Parnate)

2. Antipsychotics

Used primarily to manage psychosis (including delusions, hallucinations, paranoia or disordered thought), which can occur in disorders like schizophrenia and bipolar disorder. Antipsychotics can also be used at lower doses to treat anxiety and depression.

- **Typical Antipsychotics**: e.g., Haloperidol (Haldol), Chlorpromazine (Thorazine)

- **Atypical Antipsychotics**: e.g., Risperidone (Risperdal), Olanzapine (Zyprexa), Quetiapine (Seroquel), Aripiprazole (Abilify)

3. Mood Stabilizers

Used to treat bipolar disorder, mood stabilizers help even out the highs (manic episodes) and lows (depressive episodes) associated with the condition.

- **Lithium** (often considered a class of its own)

- **Anticonvulsants**: e.g., Valproate (Depakote), Lamotrigine (Lamictal), Carbamazepine (Tegretol)

4. Anxiolytics

These medications are used to relieve anxiety. They are typically prescribed for short-term use due to the risk of dependence.

- **Benzodiazepines**: e.g., Diazepam (Valium), Alprazolam (Xanax), Lorazepam (Ativan)

- **Buspirone** (often used for chronic anxiety without the risk of dependence associated with benzodiazepines)

5. Stimulants

Primarily used to treat attention-deficit hyperactivity disorder (ADHD), stimulants enhance concentration and focus while reducing hyperactive and impulsive behavior.

- **Amphetamines**: e.g., Adderall, Dextroamphetamine (Dexedrine)

- **Methylphenidate**: e.g., Ritalin, Concerta

6. Central Nervous System (CNS) Depressants

Used to treat disorders such as insomnia and sleep disorders. These medications help to calm the brain activity, allowing for better sleep.

- **Z-drugs**: e.g., Zolpidem (Ambien)

- **Barbiturates**: e.g., Phenobarbital (rarely used today due to high risk of dependency and overdose)

7. Cognitive Enhancers

Used in conditions like Alzheimer's disease to help improve memory, attention, reason, language, and the ability to perform simple tasks.

- **Cholinesterase Inhibitors**: e.g., Donepezil (Aricept), Rivastigmine (Exelon)

Each of these medications comes with its own set of potential side effects and considerations for use, making it essential for healthcare providers to monitor patients closely, especially when initiating or changing a treatment regimen. Additionally, patient education on medication use, possible side effects, and the importance of adherence to prescribed therapy is critical in the management of mental health conditions.

Guidelines for administering and monitoring medication

Administering and monitoring medication in the treatment of mental health conditions requires meticulous attention to detail, a deep understanding of pharmacodynamics and pharmacokinetics, and a comprehensive approach to patient care. Here are some key guidelines for effectively administering and monitoring medication in mental health settings:

1. Thorough Patient Assessment

- **Initial Evaluation**: Conduct a complete medical and psychiatric history before starting any medication. Include any history of substance use, allergies, previous medication trials and responses, and family history of psychiatric disorders.

- **Physical Examination**: Some medications require baseline vital signs, weight, and possibly other physical examinations or laboratory tests (e.g., liver function tests for patients prescribed certain antipsychotics or mood stabilizers).

2. Informed Consent

- **Education**: Educate patients about the purposes, potential benefits, and risks of a medication, including common and serious side effects.

- **Decision-making**: Ensure that the patient is involved in the decision-making process, empowering them to make informed choices about their treatment.

3. Medication Administration

- **Adherence to Prescriptions**: Administer medications exactly as prescribed, regarding both dosage and timing.

- **Documentation**: Keep meticulous records of all medications administered, including the date, time, dosage, and any immediate reactions or side effects noted.

- **Monitoring for Interactions**: Be aware of possible drug interactions with other medications the patient may be taking, including over-the-counter medications and herbal supplements.

4. Monitoring and Managing Side Effects

- **Regular Monitoring**: Routinely monitor patients for side effects and therapeutic responses. For some medications, this might include periodic blood tests to monitor blood levels of the medication or its effects on organs (e.g., lithium levels, liver enzymes).

- **Proactive Management**: Address side effects proactively by adjusting dosages, changing medications, or prescribing additional treatments to mitigate side effects.

5. Ongoing Assessment of Medication Efficacy

- **Therapeutic Monitoring**: Regularly assess the medication's effectiveness in achieving the desired therapeutic outcomes.

- **Adjustments**: Be prepared to adjust dosages or change medications as necessary, based on the patient's response and any side effects they experience.

6. Patient and Family Education

- **Understanding Medication**: Ensure that both the patient and their family understand why the medication is being prescribed, how to take it properly, and the importance of adherence to the regimen.

- **Awareness of Side Effects**: Educate on how to recognize serious side effects and the importance of reporting them immediately.

7. Communication with Other Healthcare Providers

- **Coordination of Care**: Maintain open lines of communication with other healthcare providers involved in the patient's care, including primary care physicians, psychiatrists, and therapists, to ensure a coordinated approach to medication management.

- **Information Sharing**: Share important information about the patient's medication regimen, response, and any side effects with all members of the healthcare team.

8. Use of Technology

- **Electronic Health Records (EHR)**: Utilize EHRs to improve the accuracy of medication records, enhance the tracking of patient progress, and facilitate the secure sharing of patient information among providers.

- **Medication Management Apps**: Encourage patients to use medication management apps to help them remember to take their medications and track their side effects.

9. Legal and Ethical Considerations

- **Ethical Standards**: Follow ethical standards and local regulations regarding medication administration, protecting patient privacy and confidentiality at all times.

- **Reportable Events**: Be aware of and report any medication errors or adverse reactions according to institutional policies and regulatory requirements.

Effective medication management in mental health is crucial and involves careful planning, collaboration, and continued evaluation to ensure that therapeutic goals are met while minimizing risks to the patient.

Addressing side effects and medication adherence

Addressing side effects and ensuring medication adherence are critical aspects of managing any treatment plan, especially in mental health, where medications can significantly impact a patient's quality of life and the effectiveness of treatment. Here's how healthcare providers, particularly mental health nurses, can manage these challenges effectively:

Addressing Side Effects

1. **Educate Patients and Families**

   - **Preparation**: Before starting a new medication, provide comprehensive information about potential side effects. Knowing what to expect can reduce anxiety and prevent panic if side effects occur.

   - **Empowerment**: Teach patients and their families how to recognize and report side effects promptly.

2. **Monitor Regularly**

   - **Scheduled Check-ins**: Implement regular monitoring check-ins to assess for any side effects. This could be through follow-up appointments, telephone calls, or digital health platforms.

   - **Use of Tools**: Encourage patients to keep a diary of their symptoms and any side effects, which can be useful for identifying patterns or triggers.

3. **Proactive Management**

- **Adjustment of Dosage**: If side effects are mild, adjusting the dosage may alleviate them without compromising the effectiveness of the treatment.

- **Switching Medications**: For more severe side effects, consider transitioning to a different medication. This should be done cautiously and under close supervision.

4. **Symptom Management**

- **Supportive Care**: Provide or recommend additional treatments or remedies to manage symptoms (e.g., anti-nausea medication for patients experiencing nausea due to antidepressants).

Enhancing Medication Adherence

1. **Simplify the Regimen**

- **Fewer Doses**: Whenever possible, prescribe medications that require fewer daily doses to simplify the regimen.

- **Combination Pills**: Use combination medications that address multiple symptoms in one pill to reduce the number of medications a patient must take.

2. **Education and Communication**

- **Understanding Benefits**: Ensure that patients understand how the medications help with their condition, reinforcing the benefits of staying on medication as prescribed.

- **Open Communication**: Foster an environment where patients feel comfortable discussing their struggles with medication, including any desires to stop due to side effects or perceived lack of efficacy.

3. **Use of Reminders and Support Tools**

- **Technology Aids**: Recommend the use of apps or digital alerts to remind patients when to take their medication.

- **Support Systems**: Involve family members or caregivers in the treatment plan, where appropriate, to help support the patient's medication regimen.

4. **Behavioral Techniques**

- **Motivational Interviewing**: Use motivational interviewing techniques to enhance motivation and commitment to the treatment regimen.

- **Problem-Solving**: Help patients identify and overcome barriers to adherence (e.g., financial issues, forgetfulness).

5. **Regular Follow-Up**

- **Continuous Monitoring**: Regular follow-up appointments can help keep patients accountable and provide opportunities to discuss and reassess the treatment plan.

- **Adjustments as Needed**: Be willing to make adjustments to the treatment plan based on patient feedback and clinical outcomes.

6. **Address Financial and Access Issues**

- **Cost Management**: Assist patients in finding ways to manage costs, such as using generic drugs, applying for patient assistance programs, or exploring insurance coverage options.

- **Pharmacy Coordination**: Coordinate with pharmacies to use automatic refills to ease the burden on patients.

By implementing these strategies, mental health professionals can help manage side effects effectively and improve medication adherence, leading to better health outcomes and enhanced patient satisfaction.

Chapter 5: Legal and Ethical Issues in Mental Health Nursing

Understanding patient rights and nurse responsibilities

Understanding patient rights and nurse responsibilities is crucial in fostering a respectful, ethical, and legally compliant healthcare environment. In the context of mental health care, where patients may be particularly vulnerable, it is essential to emphasize these aspects to ensure the dignity, safety, and well-being of patients are upheld.

Patient Rights in Mental Health Care

1. **Right to Informed Consent**

   - Patients have the right to receive clear and comprehensive information about their diagnosis, treatment options, potential risks, and benefits in a manner they can understand. This enables them to make informed decisions about their care.

2. **Right to Privacy and Confidentiality**

   - Patient information must be kept confidential and shared only with those directly involved in their care or as mandated by law. Patients also have the right to access their medical records.

3. **Right to Respect and Dignity**

- Every patient deserves to be treated with respect and dignity, regardless of their mental health condition. This includes respectful communication, consideration of personal preferences, and recognition of individuality.

4. **Right to Safety**

- Patients have the right to receive care in a safe environment free from abuse, harm, and neglect. This includes the right to be free from physical restraints or seclusion unless absolutely necessary for safety.

5. **Right to Participate in Their Care**

- Patients have the right to be involved in all aspects of their care, including the development and updates of their treatment plans. This also encompasses the right to refuse treatment, except in situations where they may pose a danger to themselves or others.

6. **Right to Communication**

- Patients have the right to communicate freely with people outside the hospital and to receive visitors within reasonable limits and conditions.

7. **Right to Least Restrictive Care**

- Mental health care should be delivered in the least restrictive environment necessary to meet the patient's needs, promoting freedom and autonomy as much as possible.

Nurse Responsibilities in Mental Health Care

1. **Advocacy**

   - Nurses must advocate for the rights and best interests of their patients, ensuring they receive appropriate care and their rights are respected.

2. **Providing Informed Consent**

   - It is the nurse's responsibility to ensure that patients or their legal representatives receive all necessary information in a digestible format to make informed healthcare decisions.

3. **Ensuring Confidentiality**

   - Nurses are responsible for safeguarding patient information, sharing it only with authorized individuals as necessary for patient care or under legal requirements.

4. **Respect and Dignity**

   - Nurses must treat all patients with respect and dignity, acknowledging their value and rights as individuals, and accommodate their cultural, spiritual, and personal values.

5. **Safety and Quality Care**

- Nurses are responsible for providing safe, high-quality care. This includes using evidence-based practices and interventions, performing regular risk assessments, and taking immediate action to address potential safety issues.

6. **Education and Support**

- Educating patients about their conditions, treatment options, and prevention measures is a key nursing responsibility. Providing emotional support and guidance throughout the treatment process is also crucial.

7. **Professional Competence**

- Nurses must maintain professional competence through ongoing education and training, ensuring their practices meet current standards of care.

By upholding these patient rights and fulfilling their responsibilities, nurses not only enhance the quality of mental health care but also foster trust and therapeutic relationships with their patients, leading to better health outcomes and patient satisfaction.

Dealing with ethical dilemmas in mental health care

Dealing with ethical dilemmas in mental health care is a complex and sensitive aspect of practice, requiring careful consideration and a balance of various ethical principles.

Mental health professionals often encounter situations where the right course of action isn't clear-cut, necessitating a structured approach to decision-making. Here are some common ethical dilemmas in mental health care and strategies for addressing them effectively:

Common Ethical Dilemmas

1. **Confidentiality vs. the Need to Warn**

   - Dilemma: When a patient discloses information that suggests a serious risk to others, professionals face a conflict between maintaining patient confidentiality and the duty to warn potential victims.

   - Example: A patient expresses specific threats towards an individual or group.

2. **Involuntary Treatment**

   - Dilemma: Deciding when to override a patient's autonomy to ensure their safety or the safety of others, such as in cases of severe mental illness where the patient refuses treatment but poses a risk.

   - Example: A patient with severe psychosis refuses medication, believing it is poison, but is gravely disabled by their illness.

3. **Patient Competence**

   - Dilemma: Assessing a patient's capacity to make decisions about their own care, particularly in fluctuating conditions like bipolar disorder or dementia.

- Example: A patient with bipolar disorder in a manic phase wants to make significant financial decisions.

4. **Resource Allocation**

- Dilemma: Balancing the equitable distribution of limited mental health resources, such as deciding who receives access to specialized programs or treatments.

- Example: Prioritizing patients for a limited number of beds in a treatment facility.

Strategies for Addressing Ethical Dilemmas

1. **Ethical Decision-Making Frameworks**

- Utilize structured frameworks to analyze and make decisions regarding ethical dilemmas. Common frameworks include the four-box method (medical indications, patient preferences, quality of life, and contextual features) or the use of ethical principles such as autonomy, beneficence, non-maleficence, and justice.

2. **Consultation and Collaboration**

- Engage with colleagues, ethics committees, or multidisciplinary teams to gather diverse perspectives and expertise. Collaborative discussions can provide insights and alternative solutions that may not be apparent individually.

3. **Legal Guidance**

- Consult legal precedents and statutes related to mental health care, especially concerning involuntary treatment and duty to warn. Understanding legal obligations can help clarify the limits and obligations of ethical practice.

4. **Patient and Family Engagement**

- Involve patients and their families in discussions about care whenever possible. This engagement is crucial for respecting patient autonomy and making informed decisions that consider the patient's values and preferences.

5. **Documentation**

- Document all decisions thoroughly, including the rationale behind each decision and the discussions that led to it. Documentation should reflect the ethical considerations, clinical judgments, and patient or family inputs.

6. **Education and Training**

- Regularly participate in ethics training and education to stay informed about emerging issues and effective approaches to ethical dilemmas in mental health care. Continuous learning can help anticipate and navigate complex situations more effectively.

7. **Emotional Support for Staff**

- Recognize the emotional toll that ethical dilemmas can have on health care providers. Support systems such as supervision, counseling, and peer support groups are essential for maintaining professional integrity and emotional resilience.

Addressing ethical dilemmas in mental health care involves a careful balance of respecting patient rights, ensuring safety, and adhering to legal and professional standards. By systematically applying ethical principles and engaging in collaborative decision-making, mental health professionals can navigate these challenges with confidence and care.

Confidentiality, consent, and legal considerations

Confidentiality, consent, and legal considerations are foundational elements in the practice of mental health care. These principles not only uphold the ethics of medical practice but also safeguard the rights and welfare of patients. Understanding and properly implementing these aspects are crucial for building trust, ensuring compliance with laws, and delivering high-quality care.

Confidentiality

Principle: Confidentiality involves keeping personal and medical information private and sharing it only with those who are authorized to know. In mental health, where sensitive information is often disclosed in a therapeutic setting, maintaining confidentiality is critical.

Challenges: Challenges arise when patient information needs to be disclosed under specific circumstances, such as potential harm to the patient or others (duty to warn), legal requirements (court orders), or in cases involving minors where parents or guardians might need to be informed.

Implementation:

- **Clear Communication**: Patients should be informed about the limits of confidentiality at the outset of their care.

- **Secure Information Handling**: Ensure that all patient information is stored securely and accessed only by authorized personnel.

- **Ethical Dilemmas**: Regularly consult with colleagues or ethics committees when uncertain about the appropriateness of breaking confidentiality.

Consent

Principle: Consent in mental health care involves patients giving informed agreement to receive treatment after being fully informed of the nature, consequences, and risks involved, as well as alternative treatments.

Challenges: Assessing competence to consent is a significant issue, particularly with patients who have cognitive impairments or severe mental health disorders that might impact their decision-making capacity.

Implementation:

- **Capacity Assessments**: Regularly assess the patient's capacity to understand the information necessary to make an informed decision.

- **Documentation**: Consent should always be documented, detailing the information provided to the patient and their expressed understanding and agreement.

- **Dynamic Process**: Consent is not a one-time event but a continuous process, requiring reaffirmation and reassessment, particularly when treatment plans change or new information becomes available.

Legal Considerations

Overview: Legal considerations in mental health care include complying with laws and regulations related to treatment, confidentiality, and the rights of patients. This includes understanding statutes that govern mental health practices at local, state, and federal levels.

Key Areas:

- **Mandatory Reporting**: Be aware of and comply with mandatory reporting laws, which may require

professionals to report certain conditions or
threats to the appropriate authorities.

- **Civil Commitment Laws**: Understand the laws
  related to involuntary commitment for treatment,
  which vary significantly by jurisdiction but generally
  require demonstrations of imminent danger to self
  or others.

- **Telehealth**: Adherence to legal standards regarding
  the practice of telehealth, especially concerning
  privacy laws (like HIPAA in the U.S.) and licensure
  across state lines.

Implementation:

- **Legal Consultation**: Regular consultation with legal
  professionals who specialize in health law can help
  navigate complex cases and ensure compliance
  with relevant statutes.

- **Professional Development**: Stay updated on
  changes in laws affecting mental health practice
  through continuous education and professional
  development.

By adhering to these principles and practices, mental
health professionals can protect themselves legally and
ethically, while providing safe and effective care to their
patients. It's essential to balance these considerations
carefully to maintain the integrity of the therapeutic
relationship and the efficacy of the treatment provided.

Chapter 6: Case Management and Care Planning

Steps in developing effective care plans

Developing effective care plans in mental health is a critical process that ensures each patient receives individualized, comprehensive, and coordinated care tailored to their specific needs. Here are the essential steps in developing these care plans:

1. Comprehensive Assessment

- **Gathering Information**: Collect detailed information about the patient's physical health, mental health history, social background, family history, and any current symptoms or issues. This includes using assessment tools, interviews with the patient and family, and previous medical records.

- **Identifying Needs**: Determine the patient's needs based on the assessment. This should cover a wide range of areas, including medical, psychological, social, occupational, and legal needs.

2. Setting Goals

- **Collaborative Goal Setting**: Work with the patient (and possibly their family or caregivers) to set realistic, measurable, and meaningful goals. Goals should be specific and time-bound, and they should address both short-term and long-term needs.

- **Prioritizing Goals**: Determine which goals are most urgent or have the potential to provide the most significant benefit to the patient's quality of life and begin addressing those first.

3. Planning Interventions

- **Individualized Interventions**: Based on the goals, plan specific interventions. These might include medical treatments, psychotherapy, social support, education, and changes in lifestyle or environment.

- **Evidence-Based Practices**: Use interventions supported by clinical evidence and best practices in the field of mental health.

- **Resource Allocation**: Consider what resources are available, including human resources (e.g., therapists, nurses, social workers) and material resources (e.g., medications, therapeutic materials).

4. Implementing the Plan

- **Action Steps**: Break down each intervention into actionable steps that are clear and manageable.

- **Roles and Responsibilities**: Define who is responsible for each part of the care plan, including the patient, healthcare professionals, and family members or caregivers.

- **Communication**: Ensure that everyone involved in the care understands their roles and the goals of the treatment. Effective communication is crucial to coordinate efforts and maintain consistency in approaches.

5. Monitoring and Re-evaluation

- **Regular Reviews**: Schedule regular intervals to review the progress of the care plan. This might be weekly, monthly, or quarterly, depending on the case's complexity and the interventions' nature.

- **Adjustments**: Be prepared to adjust the care plan based on the patient's progress and any new information that becomes available. Flexibility is key to responding to changes in the patient's condition or circumstances.

- **Feedback**: Incorporate feedback from the patient and other team members into the re-evaluation process to ensure that the plan remains relevant and effective.

6. Documentation

- **Record Keeping**: Document all aspects of the care plan, including assessments, goals, interventions, progress notes, and any changes made to the plan. Good documentation is essential for continuity of care, particularly if multiple providers are involved.

7. Patient and Family Education

- **Educating Patients and Families**: Educate the patient and their family about the diagnosis, the nature of the illness, treatment options, and what to expect in the treatment process. Understanding promotes better engagement and adherence to the treatment plan.

8. Support and Advocacy

- **Ongoing Support**: Provide continuous support to the patient throughout the implementation of the care plan. Support can also involve connecting the patient with community resources or advocacy services.

- **Empowerment**: Empower patients by involving them actively in their care. This increases their autonomy and encourages self-management of their condition.

Effective care planning is a dynamic, ongoing process that adapts to the evolving needs of the patient. By meticulously following these steps, mental health professionals can ensure that care plans are not only comprehensive and personalized but also implemented successfully to achieve the best possible outcomes for their patients.

Multidisciplinary approach in mental health care

A multidisciplinary approach in mental health care involves a team of health professionals from various fields working collaboratively to provide comprehensive treatment to patients. This approach is crucial because mental health conditions often affect and are influenced by multiple aspects of a person's health and life. By integrating the expertise of various specialists, the care plan can address these multifaceted needs more effectively.

Key Components of a Multidisciplinary Approach

1. Diverse Expertise

- The team may include **psychiatrists**, who provide medical and pharmacological management; **clinical psychologists** and **psychotherapists**, who offer psychological assessments and therapy; **social workers**, who assist with social and environmental issues; **nurses**, who manage day-to-day care and monitoring; **occupational therapists**, who help improve daily functioning; and specialists like **dietitians** or **physical therapists** if needed.

2. Comprehensive Assessment

- Each professional contributes their expertise to a comprehensive assessment, helping to build a complete picture of the patient's physical, mental, and social health. This holistic view is essential for effective treatment planning.

3. Integrated Care Plan

- The team collaborates to develop an integrated care plan that addresses all aspects of the patient's health. This plan includes medical treatments, psychological therapies, social interventions, and any other necessary support services.

4. Regular Communication

- Effective communication among team members is vital. Regular team meetings ensure that all members are updated on the patient's progress and can adjust the treatment plan as needed. This coordination helps to provide consistent and cohesive care.

5. Patient and Family Involvement

- Patients and their families are often considered part of the team. Their input and feedback are crucial in setting realistic goals and making decisions about the treatment plan. This involvement also helps in educating them about the condition, treatment options, and expected outcomes, which can improve treatment adherence and effectiveness.

Benefits of a Multidisciplinary Approach

1. Holistic Care

- Patients receive care that is tailored to all their needs, not just their psychiatric symptoms. This can improve overall outcomes, as mental health is closely linked to physical health and social well-being.

2. Enhanced Expertise

- With specialists from various fields involved, the care plan benefits from a broader range of expertise. This can be particularly important for complex cases where different aspects of the person's health are affected.

3. Improved Treatment Adherence

- When patients are involved in their care planning and have support from various professionals, they are often more motivated to adhere to the treatment recommendations. This engagement can lead to better health outcomes.

4. Early Identification and Intervention

- A team of professionals can more readily identify potential complications or new issues as they arise. Early intervention can prevent problems from worsening.

5. Continuity of Care

- Having a team in place can help ensure continuity of care, especially in settings where a patient might otherwise see many different healthcare providers. This consistency is crucial for building trust and for effective long-term management of mental health conditions.

Implementing a multidisciplinary approach can be complex, requiring coordination, communication, and resources, but the benefits for patient care and outcomes in mental health settings make it a highly valuable model. This approach not only enhances the quality of care provided but also supports the professionals involved through shared responsibilities and insights.

Case studies to illustrate care planning processes

Case studies are valuable educational tools that illustrate the complexities and application of care planning processes in mental health settings. They provide insight into the decision-making process, the coordination of a multidisciplinary team, and the effectiveness of individualized care plans. Here are two hypothetical case studies that explore these aspects in mental health care:

Case Study 1: Managing Major Depressive Disorder

Background:

- **Patient**: John, a 45-year-old male

- **Presenting Problem**: John has been experiencing persistent sadness, loss of interest in daily activities, significant weight loss, insomnia, and recurring thoughts of death for the past six months.

Assessment:

- Conducted by a multidisciplinary team including a psychiatrist, a clinical psychologist, and a mental health nurse.

- Assessment findings confirmed major depressive disorder, moderate severity, without psychotic features.

Care Planning:

- **Goals**: To reduce symptoms of depression, improve sleep quality, and enhance overall functioning.

- **Interventions**:

    - **Medical**: Psychiatrist prescribes an SSRI antidepressant and schedules regular follow-ups to monitor side effects and effectiveness.

    - **Psychotherapy**: Clinical psychologist begins weekly cognitive-behavioral therapy (CBT) sessions to address negative thought patterns.

    - **Supportive Nursing Care**: Mental health nurse provides education on medication adherence, side effect management, and strategies for improving sleep hygiene.

    - **Social Support**: Referral to a community support group for individuals with depression.

Outcome:

- After three months, John reports a significant improvement in mood and motivation. He continues to attend CBT sessions and participates actively in his community support group. Medication adjustments were made in the initial weeks to optimize dosing with minimal side effects.

Reflection:

- This case illustrates the importance of a coordinated approach involving medication, therapy, and community support, highlighting the role of each team member in the patient's recovery.

Case Study 2: Addressing Schizophrenia with Comorbid Substance Use

Background:

- **Patient**: Emily, a 30-year-old female

- **Presenting Problem**: Diagnosed with schizophrenia and recently began exhibiting increased paranoia and auditory hallucinations. Also reports increased alcohol use as a coping mechanism.

Assessment:

- Comprehensive evaluation by a psychiatrist, a clinical psychologist, an addiction specialist, and a mental health nurse.

- Identified worsening of schizophrenia symptoms and risky levels of alcohol consumption.

Care Planning:

- **Goals**: To stabilize psychiatric symptoms, achieve sobriety, and integrate coping strategies for stress management.

- **Interventions**:

  - **Medical**: Psychiatrist adjusts antipsychotic medication and integrates a medication to reduce alcohol craving.

- **Dual Diagnosis Treatment**: Addiction specialist provides counseling focused on substance abuse and its impact on schizophrenia.

- **Psychotherapy**: Clinical psychologist works on cognitive-behavioral strategies to manage paranoia and hallucinations.

- **Nursing Support**: Mental health nurse oversees the daily management of medication regimes, monitors for side effects, and provides regular health education.

Outcome:

- Six months later, Emily has achieved sobriety and reports a reduction in paranoia and hallucinations. She continues to engage in regular therapy sessions and has joined a support group for individuals with dual diagnoses.

Reflection:

- Emily's case underscores the complexity of treating schizophrenia with comorbid substance use, demonstrating how tailored interventions from a multidisciplinary team can address diverse aspects of a patient's health.

These case studies show how structured care planning involving a multidisciplinary team can effectively address the multifaceted needs of mental health patients, ensuring comprehensive care that enhances their path to recovery.

Chapter 7: Crisis Intervention and Acute Care

Recognizing mental health crises

Recognizing a mental health crisis is critical for timely and effective intervention. Mental health crises can vary widely, but they generally involve situations where an individual's behavior poses a significant risk to themselves or others, or they are unable to function in daily life due to acute psychological distress. Here are key signs and symptoms to help identify a mental health crisis and the appropriate steps to address it:

Key Signs of a Mental Health Crisis

1. **Extreme Mood Swings**: Significant, rapid shifts in mood that are unusual for the person.

2. **Agitation or Aggression**: Noticeable increase in irritability, hostility, or aggressive behavior that is not characteristic of the individual's usual behavior.

3. **Withdrawal**: Severe withdrawal from social interaction, daily activities, or responsibilities, especially if this is a marked change.

4. **Psychotic Symptoms**: This includes hallucinations (seeing or hearing things that aren't there) or delusions (persistent beliefs in things that are not true or based in reality).

5. **Paranoia or Anxiety**: Heightened paranoia or anxiety that is debilitating and interferes with daily functioning.

6. **Expressing Suicidal Thoughts**: Any talk about suicide, dying, or self-harm should be taken very seriously, particularly if the person is expressing a plan or intent.

7. **Substance Abuse**: Sudden increase in substance use or using substances as a way to cope with emotional distress.

8. **Inability to Perform Daily Tasks**: Demonstrating an inability to sleep, eat, maintain personal hygiene, or perform other basic activities.

Steps to Address a Mental Health Crisis

1. **Stay Calm and Assure Safety**: Approach the person in a calm and reassuring manner. Ensure the environment is safe for both the individual and others nearby.

2. **Communicate Effectively**: Use clear, simple, and direct communication. Listen actively and empathetically without dismissing the person's feelings.

3. **Assess the Severity**: Quickly assess the level of risk. Determine if the individual is in immediate danger to themselves or others. Look for signs of potential self-harm or suicide, and check if they have access to means (like weapons or drugs).

4. **Provide Support**: Express your concern and willingness to help. Let them know that they are not alone and that there is help available. Avoid challenging or arguing with delusional thoughts if they are present, as this may increase agitation.

5. **Encourage Professional Help**: If the crisis is not life-threatening, encourage the individual to seek help from a mental health professional. Offer to accompany them to a mental health service or hospital if necessary.

6. **Contact Emergency Services**: If there is an immediate risk of harm to the individual or others, do not hesitate to call emergency services. Provide them with all the necessary information about the situation, including any known mental health history.

7. **Follow Up**: After the crisis has been managed, follow up with the individual to ensure they have accessed ongoing support. Continuity of care is crucial for recovery.

Training and Preparedness

- **Training**: It is advisable for anyone who might encounter individuals in crisis, such as educators, healthcare providers, and community workers, to receive training in crisis intervention techniques such as Mental Health First Aid.

- **Crisis Intervention Teams**: In many areas, there are specialized crisis intervention teams (CITs) that involve trained law enforcement officers who collaborate with mental health professionals. Knowing how to contact these teams can be vital.

Recognizing and responding effectively to mental health crises can prevent harm and ensure that individuals get the necessary care and support. Being prepared and knowledgeable about what to do in a crisis can save lives and help maintain the safety and well-being of everyone involved.

Immediate interventions and long-term strategies

In mental health care, addressing crises effectively requires both immediate interventions and long-term strategies. The goal of immediate interventions is to stabilize the situation and ensure safety, while long-term strategies focus on preventing future crises and promoting sustained mental health. Here's how these approaches can be implemented:

Immediate Interventions

1. **Ensure Safety**: The first priority in any crisis is to ensure the safety of the individual and others around them. Remove any potential means of harm, and if necessary, call emergency services to secure professional help immediately.

2. **Calm and Reassure**: Approach the person in a calm, non-threatening manner. Speak softly and reassuringly, maintaining a non-confrontational posture to help de-escalate tension.

3. **Active Listening**: Give the person your full attention. Listen without judgment to understand their feelings and needs. Acknowledging their distress without offering quick fixes can be very supportive.

4. **Assess the Situation**: Quickly assess the severity of the crisis. Determine whether the person poses a danger to themselves or others, and assess their mental and emotional state. This may dictate whether additional professional help is needed.

5. **Encourage Professional Help**: If the person is not already connected with mental health services, encourage them to seek help. Offer to assist with making appointments or finding appropriate services.

6. **Provide Immediate Support Options**: Depending on the nature of the crisis, you might offer strategies such as breathing exercises, grounding techniques, or even walking in a quiet place to help mitigate feelings of panic or overwhelming emotion.

7. **Crisis Plan**: If the person has a pre-existing mental health condition, refer to any existing crisis intervention plans. This might include contacting a mental health professional, a trusted friend, or a family member who is part of their support system.

Long-Term Strategies

1. **Comprehensive Treatment Plan**: Work with healthcare providers to develop or revise a comprehensive treatment plan that addresses the underlying causes of the crisis. This plan may include medication, therapy, and support services.

2. **Regular Follow-up**: Ensure that the person has regular follow-ups as part of their ongoing care. Continuous monitoring can help adjust treatment plans as needed and provide early intervention if another crisis appears likely.

3. **Therapy**: Long-term psychological therapy can be beneficial. Therapies such as cognitive-behavioral therapy (CBT), dialectical behavior therapy (DBT), or other modalities can help the person develop coping strategies and address the root causes of their distress.

4. **Support Networks**: Encourage the development of personal support networks, including friends, family, support groups, or community resources. Social support is vital for long-term mental health stability.

5. **Education**: Educate the individual and their support network about the signs of impending crises and effective coping mechanisms. Knowledge and preparation can prevent a crisis or lessen its severity.

6. **Lifestyle Adjustments**: Encourage healthy lifestyle changes such as regular physical activity, a balanced diet, adequate sleep, and mindfulness or

relaxation techniques, all of which can improve overall mental health.

7. **Develop a Safety Plan**: Together with the person and their mental health professionals, develop a safety plan that includes signs that indicate they are becoming unwell, coping strategies, and steps to take if they enter a crisis state again.

Implementing these immediate and long-term strategies can help stabilize individuals during a mental health crisis and significantly reduce the likelihood of future crises. These approaches promote recovery, resilience, and well-being, contributing to a higher quality of life for individuals dealing with mental health issues.

Safety considerations and emergency care procedures

In mental health care, ensuring safety and implementing appropriate emergency care procedures are vital for protecting both the individual experiencing a mental health crisis and those around them. Here are essential safety considerations and emergency care procedures to follow:

Safety Considerations

1. **Environment Safety**:

   • **Secure Environment**: Remove objects that could be used for self-harm or harm to others. Ensure the environment is calm and free of unnecessary stressors.

- **Privacy and Comfort**: Provide a private space where the individual feels safe to express themselves without fear of judgment or exposure.

2. **Staff Safety**:

- **Training**: Ensure all staff are trained in crisis intervention techniques and can recognize the early signs of agitation or aggression.

- **Team Approach**: Never deal with high-risk situations alone. Ensure there is a system for calling for immediate assistance from other staff members if needed.

3. **Patient Dignity**:

- Respect the individual's personal space and dignity during interventions. Avoid physical restraint unless absolutely necessary to prevent harm, and even then, only trained personnel should apply such measures following established protocols.

Emergency Care Procedures

1. **Initial Assessment**:

- **Evaluate the Risk**: Quickly assess the level of threat to the individual or others. Determine whether the individual is at risk of harming themselves or others.

- **Medical Evaluation**: Assess for any medical issues that may be influencing the individual's mental state, such as intoxication, withdrawal, or metabolic disturbances.

2. **De-escalation Techniques**:

   - **Communication**: Use calm, non-threatening verbal communication to engage the individual. Speak slowly and clearly, using the individual's name if known.

   - **Non-Verbal Cues**: Maintain non-threatening body language. Keep your own hands visible and avoid sudden movements.

3. **Crisis Intervention Plan**:

   - **Follow Existing Plans**: If the individual has a pre-established crisis plan, follow it as closely as possible. This may include contacting family members, their mental health provider, or a designated crisis response team.

   - **Emergency Contacts**: Have access to a list of emergency contact numbers, including crisis hotlines, local emergency services, and contacts of significant others as provided by the individual.

4. **Use of Restraints (if absolutely necessary)**:

- **Last Resort**: Restraints should only be used when less intrusive measures have failed and the person poses a clear and immediate risk to themselves or others.

- **Follow Protocols**: Use the least restrictive form of restraint and ensure it is applied correctly by trained personnel. Continuously monitor the individual's physical and psychological status during restraint.

5. **Documentation**:

- **Thorough Recording**: Document all observations, actions taken, and the individual's response to interventions. Include timing, staff involved, and any changes in the individual's condition.

6. **Transport to Healthcare Facility**:

- **Professional Transport**: If the situation escalates beyond the capability of on-site management, or if it is deemed that the individual requires psychiatric evaluation, arrange for transport to a healthcare facility. Use medical transport services if available, especially if the individual is highly agitated or poses a risk.

7. **Post-Incident Review**:

- **Staff Debriefing**: Conduct a debriefing session with all involved staff to review the incident, discuss what was effective, and identify areas for improvement.

- **Support for Affected Individuals**: Offer support to all affected, including the individual in crisis, other clients, and staff. Consider providing access to counseling services if needed.

By following these safety considerations and emergency care procedures, mental health care providers can manage crises effectively while minimizing harm and supporting the dignity and rights of the individual in crisis.

Chapter 8: Community Mental Health Nursing

Role of nurses in community settings

Nurses in community settings play a vital role in improving public health, preventing disease, and providing care and education outside of traditional hospital environments. Their responsibilities in these roles are diverse, encompassing direct patient care, education, advocacy, and coordination of services. Here's a detailed look at the various functions and impact of nurses in community settings:

Direct Care Provision

1. **Home Health Care**: Nurses provide essential medical services in patients' homes. They manage chronic conditions, administer medications, provide wound care, and offer support for family members caring for individuals with disabilities or chronic illnesses.

2. **School Nursing**: School nurses address the health needs of children and adolescents in educational settings. They manage acute illnesses, administer medications, perform screenings, and handle emergencies. They also play a critical role in managing chronic conditions such as asthma, diabetes, and allergies to ensure that children can participate fully in school activities.

3. **Elder Care**: Nurses in community settings often focus on geriatric care, providing health services in

97

residential homes or through community clinics. They monitor health, manage chronic diseases, and educate older adults and their caregivers on maintaining health and independence.

Preventive Care and Health Promotion

1. **Immunizations and Screenings**: Nurses administer vaccines and conduct routine screenings for health issues such as hypertension, diabetes, and cancer. These activities are crucial for preventing disease outbreaks and promoting early detection of health conditions.

2. **Health Education**: Community nurses provide education on nutrition, exercise, sexual health, substance abuse prevention, and chronic disease management. By offering workshops and seminars, they empower individuals and communities to take control of their health.

3. **Public Health Campaigns**: Nurses participate in public health campaigns to raise awareness about important health issues, such as smoking cessation, mental health, maternal health, and infectious disease prevention.

Advocacy and Community Engagement

1. **Policy Advocacy**: Nurses advocate for health policy changes that promote better community health outcomes. This might involve lobbying for more comprehensive healthcare services or for changes in laws affecting public health.

2. **Community Outreach**: Nurses build relationships within communities to better understand their health needs and to develop trust. This engagement facilitates more effective delivery of health services and ensures that interventions are culturally sensitive and appropriate.

3. **Resource Navigation**: Nurses help individuals and families navigate health and social services available in the community. This includes assisting with access to healthcare, social services, housing, and food assistance programs.

Coordination and Collaboration

1. **Case Management**: Nurses often serve as case managers, coordinating care for patients with complex health needs. They ensure that all aspects of a patient's care are addressed effectively, involving various health specialists as needed.

2. **Interdisciplinary Collaboration**: Community nurses work closely with physicians, social workers, therapists, and other healthcare professionals to provide holistic care. They ensure that care plans are executed cohesively across different services and specialties.

3. **Emergency Preparedness and Response**: Nurses play a key role in preparing for and responding to public health emergencies, such as natural disasters, pandemics, or bioterrorism events. They may help plan emergency responses, staff

emergency response units, and provide direct care during crises.

The role of nurses in community settings is expansive and dynamically adapts to the needs of the populations they serve. Their work not only impacts individual health outcomes but also enhances community well-being, proving essential to the broader health system.

Preventative strategies and outreach programs

Preventative strategies and outreach programs are essential components of public health that aim to reduce the incidence of disease, prevent health crises, and promote overall well-being in the community. These programs focus on early intervention, education, and creating supportive environments that encourage healthy lifestyles. Here's an overview of effective preventative strategies and outreach programs:

Preventative Strategies

1. **Screening and Early Detection Programs**

   - Regular screenings for diseases like cancer (breast, cervical, colorectal), hypertension, diabetes, and high cholesterol can lead to early detection and treatment, significantly improving outcomes.

   - Implement community-based screening events and mobile health clinics to reach underserved populations.

2. **Vaccination Clinics**

- Vaccinations are one of the most effective public health interventions. Organize clinics to administer vaccines for influenza, HPV, tetanus, COVID-19, and more, especially targeting at-risk populations.

3. **Health Education**

- Conduct workshops and seminars on nutrition, physical activity, mental health, substance abuse prevention, and sexual health to empower individuals with the knowledge to make healthier choices.

- Tailor education materials to meet the cultural and linguistic needs of diverse communities.

4. **Chronic Disease Management**

- Programs focused on managing chronic conditions such as diabetes, asthma, and heart disease help prevent complications through regular monitoring and education about diet, exercise, and medication adherence.

5. **Mental Health First Aid**

- Train community members in mental health first aid to increase awareness, reduce stigma, and provide initial support until professional help can be obtained.

Outreach Programs

1. **Mobile Health Services**

   - Deploy mobile health units to provide medical services, screenings, and education directly to hard-to-reach areas or populations who may not have regular access to healthcare facilities.

2. **School-Based Health Programs**

   - Implement programs in schools that educate children about healthy eating, physical activity, and mental health. School-based programs can include health screenings, dental check-ups, and counseling services.

3. **Workplace Wellness Programs**

   - Partner with employers to develop workplace health programs that encourage regular physical activity, healthy eating, and mental wellness. Programs can include health screenings, fitness classes, and seminars on stress management.

4. **Community Partnerships**

   - Collaborate with local organizations, such as YMCAs, religious institutions, and community centers, to host events and disseminate health information. These partnerships can amplify reach and impact.

5. **Substance Abuse Prevention and Treatment**

- Offer community education on the risks of substance abuse, provide resources for addiction recovery, and support preventive programs targeting youth.

6. **Home Visiting Programs for New and Expectant Mothers**

- Support new and expectant mothers through home visits by nurses or trained community health workers to promote maternal and infant health, provide parenting education, and ensure timely vaccinations.

7. **Telehealth Initiatives**

- Expand access to preventive care through telehealth, especially for mental health services and chronic disease management. Telehealth can be particularly beneficial in rural or underserved areas.

By implementing these preventive strategies and outreach programs, communities can significantly reduce the burden of disease, enhance the quality of life for their members, and decrease healthcare costs over time. These efforts require ongoing support, evaluation, and adaptation to meet the evolving needs of the community.

Engaging with community resources and support systems

Engaging with community resources and support systems is a fundamental aspect of comprehensive healthcare, particularly in mental health where ongoing support can significantly impact outcomes. For healthcare providers, including mental health nurses and social workers, leveraging these resources effectively can enhance treatment plans, provide necessary social support, and ensure continuity of care. Here are strategies and considerations for successfully engaging with community resources and support systems:

Identifying Community Resources

1. **Local Health Services**

   - Connect with local clinics, hospitals, and health centers that offer complementary or necessary services not provided in your primary care setting.

2. **Mental Health and Substance Abuse Services**

   - Identify specialized programs for mental health support, including counseling centers, substance abuse programs, and psychiatric services that offer both inpatient and outpatient support.

3. **Educational Programs**

   - Work with local schools and educational programs to support children and adolescents with mental health challenges. This includes special education services, school counselors, and on-site mental health professionals.

4. **Social Services**

   - Coordinate with social service agencies that can assist with housing, employment, legal aid, and food security. These services can be crucial for patients whose mental health is impacted by socio-economic factors.

5. **Support Groups and Peer Networks**

   - Encourage participation in support groups related to specific mental health issues, such as depression, anxiety, bipolar disorder, or schizophrenia. Peer support can be an invaluable resource for shared experiences and coping strategies.

6. **Recreational and Therapeutic Programs**

   - Engage with organizations that offer therapeutic activities, which might include arts and crafts centers, sports clubs, or music groups that facilitate expression and community integration.

Building Relationships

1. **Regular Communication**

   - Maintain regular contact with community organizations to stay updated on available resources, eligibility criteria, and any changes in services.

2. **Collaborative Partnerships**

- Establish formal partnerships with key community resources to streamline referrals and ensure a continuum of care for patients. This may include creating memorandums of understanding or service agreements.

3. **Cross-Training**

- Participate in or facilitate training sessions where staff from different sectors can learn about the specific needs and best practices of mental health care from each other.

Making Referrals

1. **Seamless Referral Systems**

- Develop a referral system that makes it easy for clients to access community resources. This system should include follow-up procedures to monitor the effectiveness of the referral.

2. **Personalized Referrals**

- Tailor referrals to the specific needs and circumstances of each patient. Consider their cultural, linguistic, and personal preferences to ensure the best fit.

3. **Feedback Mechanism**

- Implement a feedback mechanism to assess the patient's experience with the community resource. This feedback can guide future referrals and highlight areas for improvement in the referral process.

Advocacy

1. **Policy Advocacy**

- Advocate for policies that improve funding, access, and the quality of community resources. Engage in local health planning and policy-making committees or groups to represent mental health interests.

2. **Community Awareness Campaigns**

- Participate in or organize community awareness campaigns to educate the public about mental health, reduce stigma, and promote the resources available.

Evaluation and Adaptation

1. **Continuous Evaluation**

- Regularly evaluate the effectiveness of community engagement strategies and the impact of external resources on patient outcomes. Use this data to refine approaches and improve integration.

2. **Flexibility and Adaptation**

- Stay adaptable to changes in community resources, patient needs, and healthcare landscapes. Flexibility is key to responding effectively to new challenges and opportunities.

Engaging with community resources and support systems enriches mental health care, providing patients with comprehensive support that addresses multiple dimensions of health and well-being. By fostering robust connections with these resources, healthcare providers can enhance their capacity to deliver effective, holistic care.

Chapter 9: Addressing Stigma and Promoting Mental Health Awareness

Stigma in mental health

Stigma associated with mental health remains a significant barrier to seeking treatment, receiving adequate support, and achieving successful integration within the community. It can affect individuals experiencing mental health issues, their families, and even the healthcare providers who treat them. Understanding the impact of stigma is crucial for developing effective strategies to combat it and improve mental health outcomes.

Forms of Stigma

1. **Public Stigma**: This involves the negative or discriminatory attitudes that others have about mental illness. Public stigma can lead to prejudice, discrimination, and exclusion from various social or professional opportunities.

2. **Self-Stigma**: This occurs when individuals internalize public stigma, leading to feelings of shame, worthlessness, and a diminished sense of self-efficacy. Self-stigma can deter individuals from seeking help due to fear of being labeled or judged.

3. **Structural Stigma**: Embedded in societal institutions, this form of stigma is reflected in policies and laws that limit opportunities for people with mental health conditions. Examples include

restrictions in employment, housing, and
education.

Impact of Stigma

1. **Avoidance of Treatment**: Stigma often prevents
   individuals from seeking mental health services due
   to fear of being labeled or discriminated against.
   Delay in seeking help can lead to the worsening of
   mental health conditions.

2. **Isolation**: Individuals experiencing mental health
   issues may isolate themselves to avoid
   discrimination or out of shame associated with
   their condition. Social isolation can exacerbate
   symptoms and delay recovery.

3. **Reduced Quality of Life**: Stigma can lead to poorer
   quality of life, including difficulties in finding and
   maintaining jobs, securing housing, and
   establishing relationships. It can also affect physical
   health due to associated stress and lack of social
   support.

4. **Impacts on Family and Friends**: Families and
   friends of those with mental health issues may also
   experience stigma by association. This can lead to
   social isolation for family members and can strain
   family dynamics.

5. **Workplace Challenges**: Stigma can lead to
   discrimination in the workplace, where individuals
   may face job rejection or unfair treatment by
   employers and colleagues. This often results in

underemployment or unemployment among those with mental health conditions.

Strategies to Combat Stigma

1. **Education and Awareness**: Raising awareness about mental health issues through education can challenge myths and misconceptions. Educational campaigns should aim to inform the public about the nature of mental health conditions, the fact that they are common and treatable, and the importance of support and empathy.

2. **Personal Stories**: Encouraging individuals who have experienced mental health issues to share their stories can humanize the subject and increase empathy among the broader public. This approach helps to put a face to mental health conditions, making them more relatable.

3. **Media Representation**: Promoting accurate and sensitive representations of mental health in the media is crucial. The media has a powerful role in shaping public perceptions and can either perpetuate stigma or help to dismantle it.

4. **Supportive Policies and Legislation**: Advocating for policies that protect the rights of individuals with mental health conditions and promote equality can help reduce structural stigma. This includes laws that prevent discrimination in employment, education, and healthcare.

5. **Community Programs**: Developing community programs that promote social inclusion and provide support can help reduce isolation and empower individuals with mental health conditions. These programs can also provide platforms for engagement and education within the community.

6. **Training for Professionals**: Ensuring that healthcare providers and other professionals are trained to treat individuals with mental health conditions with respect and without prejudice is essential. Professional training should also include strategies to address one's own biases and assumptions.

By understanding and addressing the layers of stigma associated with mental health, society can move towards more inclusive and supportive attitudes, which in turn can significantly improve the health outcomes and quality of life for those affected.

Strategies for combating stigma in healthcare and communities

Combating stigma associated with mental health is essential for fostering a supportive environment that encourages individuals to seek help and to openly discuss their experiences without fear of judgment. Stigma reduction requires a coordinated effort across various sectors including healthcare, education, media, and community engagement. Here are several effective strategies for combating stigma in healthcare settings and broader communities:

In Healthcare Settings

1. **Education for Healthcare Professionals**

   - Provide ongoing training to all healthcare providers on mental health issues, emphasizing the biological and medical aspects of mental illnesses to counteract misconceptions.

   - Highlight the importance of empathy, respect, and dignity in patient care. Training should address personal biases and the impact of stigma on patient outcomes.

2. **Promote Patient-Centered Care**

   - Encourage practices that involve patients in their own care planning and decision-making processes. This empowers patients and reinforces their autonomy and dignity.

   - Ensure that communications are respectful and that patients are fully informed about their treatment options and involved in discussions about their care.

3. **Visibility and Open Discussions**

   - Create forums and panels where mental health professionals discuss mental health openly and share success stories, which can normalize mental health treatment.

   - Implement campaigns within healthcare facilities that focus on educating patients and staff about mental health, aiming to shift perceptions and encourage a more supportive environment.

In Communities

1. **Community Education and Outreach**

   - Organize workshops, seminars, and public talks on mental health that are accessible to the broader community. These should aim to educate the public about the facts of mental health conditions, treatment options, and the experiences of those affected.

   - Distribute educational materials in common community spaces like libraries, schools, religious centers, and online platforms.

2. **Engagement Through Media**

   - Collaborate with media outlets to ensure that mental health coverage is accurate, respectful, and informative. Media plays a crucial role in shaping public perceptions and can be a powerful tool in reducing stigma.

   - Support media productions that feature positive portrayals of individuals with mental health conditions, highlighting stories of recovery and effective management.

3. **Support Groups and Peer Advocates**

- Facilitate the formation of support groups where individuals can share their experiences in a safe and supportive environment. Peer support has been shown to be effective in reducing stigma by fostering a sense of community and mutual understanding.

- Train peer advocates who can speak at public events and schools, sharing their experiences and serving as real-life examples of people living successfully with mental health conditions.

4. **Policy Advocacy**

- Advocate for policies that reduce stigma and discrimination against those with mental health issues, such as laws that ensure equal rights in employment, education, and healthcare.

- Encourage local leaders to prioritize mental health services and support anti-stigma campaigns, demonstrating a community-wide commitment to addressing mental health.

5. **Community Collaborations**

- Partner with schools, workplaces, and religious institutions to integrate mental health education into their regular programming. This can include training for teachers, employers, and religious leaders on how to address mental health issues and support individuals showing signs of distress.

- Organize community events that focus on mental health awareness, such as walks, runs, or health fairs, which can help to destigmatize mental health issues and encourage community solidarity.

These strategies require a multi-faceted approach and the involvement of various stakeholders, including healthcare providers, educators, policymakers, and community leaders, to effectively combat stigma in healthcare and community settings. By working together, these groups can foster an environment where mental health is openly discussed, better understood, and more effectively supported.

Promoting mental health awareness

Promoting mental health awareness is crucial for reducing stigma, improving access to care, and enhancing the overall well-being of communities. Various initiatives and programs can be implemented to achieve these goals effectively. These efforts can vary widely in scope and scale, but all aim to educate the public, support individuals with mental health issues, and create environments that foster mental well-being. Here are some initiatives and programs that have been effective in promoting mental health awareness:

1. Public Awareness Campaigns

- **Mental Health Month**: Leverage nationally recognized months (like Mental Health Awareness Month in May in the U.S.) to organize events, share information, and highlight stories that encourage a broader understanding of mental health issues.

- **World Mental Health Day**: Participate in and promote international observances to raise awareness and mobilize efforts in support of mental health.

2. Educational Programs

- **School-based Programs**: Implement curriculum components that educate students about mental health from an early age, including how to recognize signs of mental health issues, coping mechanisms, and ways to seek help.

- **Workplace Mental Health Initiatives**: Develop programs that focus on stress management, work-life balance, and resources for mental health support within the workplace. This can include workshops, regular wellness activities, and confidential counseling services.

3. Community Workshops and Seminars

- **Free Public Workshops**: Offer workshops in community centers, libraries, or online that cover various mental health topics, including the signs of mental health issues, modern treatment options, and how to support someone who is struggling.

- **Speaker Series and Expert Panels**: Organize talks featuring mental health professionals, advocates, and individuals with lived experiences to discuss mental health openly and provide insights and education.

4. Digital and Social Media Campaigns

- **Social Media Awareness Drives**: Use platforms like Twitter, Instagram, Facebook, and YouTube to disseminate information, share stories, and connect people with resources. Social media can reach a wide audience quickly and can be particularly effective in engaging younger demographics.

- **Online Webinars and Live Sessions**: Provide interactive online learning opportunities where participants can ask questions and learn from mental health professionals.

5. Support and Advocacy Networks

- **Peer Support Networks**: Establish or support peer-led groups where individuals with similar experiences can share their stories, offer support, and advocate for better mental health policies and practices.

- **Advocacy Groups**: Collaborate with or support advocacy organizations that work towards policy changes, improved mental health services, and increased funding for mental health care.

6. Training and Certification Programs

- **Mental Health First Aid Training**: Offer training for individuals to become certified in Mental Health First Aid, teaching them how to respond in a mental health crisis and offer initial support until professional help can be obtained.

- **Professional Development**: Provide ongoing training for healthcare providers, educators, and community leaders to ensure they are equipped with up-to-date knowledge and skills to support mental health in their communities.

7. Partnerships with Healthcare Providers

- **Collaborations with Local Clinics and Hospitals**: Partner with medical institutions to provide comprehensive information and resources on mental health services available to community members.

- **Integrated Health Services**: Advocate for and support the integration of mental health services into primary healthcare settings to make mental health care more accessible.

These initiatives and programs can significantly enhance mental health awareness and literacy, helping to create a society where mental health is prioritized and effectively supported. Each community may have different needs and resources, so it's important to tailor these initiatives to fit local contexts and cultures.

Chapter 10: Case Studies in Mental Health Nursing

Real-life case studies from various mental health settings

Using real-life case studies in discussions about mental health can provide valuable insights into the complexities of diagnosis, treatment, and patient experiences. These case studies also highlight the multidisciplinary approach often necessary for effective mental health care. Below, I've outlined several hypothetical case studies drawn from various mental health settings. Each case study addresses a different aspect of mental health care, illustrating common challenges and effective interventions.

Case Study 1: Community Mental Health Center

Patient: "John", a 40-year-old male with a history of bipolar disorder.

Scenario: John was referred to a community mental health center after a severe manic episode that led to police involvement.

Intervention: John was stabilized on new medication and began regular therapy sessions. The center also involved his family in therapy sessions to educate them about bipolar disorder and how to support John's treatment.

Outcome: After six months, John reported feeling more stable and was able to return to work. His family felt more equipped to support him, and they were aware of the signs that indicated he needed additional help.

Case Study 2: Inpatient Psychiatric Facility

Patient: "Emma", a 26-year-old female diagnosed with severe depression and suicidal ideation.

Scenario: Emma was voluntarily admitted to an inpatient psychiatric facility following a suicide attempt.

Intervention: Emma participated in intensive daily individual and group therapy, including cognitive-behavioral therapy (CBT) and dialectical behavior therapy (DBT). Medication was carefully managed to address her depressive symptoms.

Outcome: Emma's condition improved significantly over a three-week stay. Upon discharge, she was linked with an outpatient psychiatrist and a therapist specializing in DBT to continue her care.

Case Study 3: School-Based Mental Health Program

Patient: "Carlos", a 15-year-old student with anxiety and panic attacks.

Scenario: Carlos was referred to the school counselor after experiencing several panic attacks at school.

Intervention: The school-based mental health program provided Carlos with counseling sessions during school hours. The counselor also worked with Carlos's teachers to develop strategies to reduce stress in the classroom.

Outcome: Carlos learned coping strategies to manage his anxiety and was able to participate more fully in class. His academic performance improved as his anxiety was better managed.

Case Study 4: Residential Treatment for Substance Abuse

Patient: "Linda", a 35-year-old female with alcohol use disorder and depression.

Scenario: Linda sought help through a residential treatment program after her drinking led to multiple hospitalizations.

Intervention: The program integrated treatment for both substance abuse and depression, involving medication, individual therapy, group support sessions, and skill-building activities.

Outcome: Linda developed a strong support network and learned strategies to manage her depression without alcohol. She continued her recovery with weekly group meetings and regular therapy sessions after leaving the residential program.

Case Study 5: Telehealth for Rural Mental Health

Patient: "Mark", a 50-year-old male living in a rural area, struggling with PTSD.

Scenario: Mark had limited access to mental health services in his area and was referred to a telehealth service by his primary care provider.

Intervention: Mark engaged in weekly video sessions with a therapist who specialized in PTSD. He was also part of a virtual support group with others facing similar challenges.

Outcome: Mark reported a decrease in PTSD symptoms and felt less isolated. The convenience of telehealth made consistent therapy possible, significantly improving his quality of life.

Case Study 6: Elderly Patient with Late-Onset Depression

Patient: "Alice", a 72-year-old female diagnosed with late-onset depression following the death of her spouse.

Scenario: Alice showed signs of persistent sadness, withdrawal from social activities, and a loss of interest in previously enjoyed hobbies.

Intervention: Alice was referred to a geriatric psychiatrist who prescribed antidepressants and initiated weekly therapy sessions. Additionally, she was encouraged to join a local senior community center to engage in social activities and grief counseling.

Outcome: Over several months, Alice reported improvements in mood and motivation. Participation in community activities provided her with a support network of peers, contributing to her overall wellbeing.

Case Study 7: Adolescent with Attention-Deficit Hyperactivity Disorder (ADHD)

Patient: "Ben", a 14-year-old male struggling with ADHD, which was affecting his academic performance and social interactions.

Scenario: Ben's teachers and parents were concerned about his inability to focus, impulsiveness, and declining academic grades.

Intervention: After a comprehensive evaluation, Ben was prescribed stimulant medication and enrolled in a behavioral therapy program. His school implemented an individualized education program (IEP) to provide additional support.

Outcome: With medication, therapy, and tailored educational support, Ben's concentration improved, and he became more engaged in school. His social relationships also benefited from the behavioral strategies he learned during therapy.

Case Study 8: Adult with Schizophrenia

Patient: "Claire", a 30-year-old female diagnosed with schizophrenia, known for experiencing auditory hallucinations and delusions.

Scenario: Claire had difficulty maintaining employment and personal relationships due to her symptoms.

Intervention: Claire was admitted to a psychiatric facility for stabilization and began a treatment regimen including antipsychotic medication and cognitive behavioral therapy tailored for psychosis. She also received social skills training.

Outcome: Claire's hallucinations and delusions became less frequent and severe, allowing her to live more independently. She continued outpatient treatment and joined a job-training program designed for individuals with mental health conditions.

Case Study 9: Veteran with Post-Traumatic Stress Disorder (PTSD)

Patient: "David", a 45-year-old military veteran experiencing PTSD characterized by severe flashbacks, nightmares, and isolation.

Scenario: David was initially reluctant to seek help due to stigma and pride.

Intervention: Encouraged by a fellow veteran, David visited a veteran's health clinic where he was introduced to a PTSD support group and began prolonged exposure therapy. He also engaged in complementary therapies, including equine therapy.

Outcome: David's engagement with therapy and the support group led to a noticeable improvement in his symptoms. His social interactions increased, and he reported feeling more hopeful about the future.

Case Study 10: Young Adult with Borderline Personality Disorder (BPD)

Patient: "Eva", a 25-year-old female diagnosed with BPD, struggling with emotional instability, impulsive behaviors, and intense episodic depression.

Scenario: Eva's relationships were highly volatile, and she had a history of self-harm.

Intervention: Eva was enrolled in a dialectical behavior therapy (DBT) program, which included both individual and group therapy sessions. This program focused on

126

teaching coping mechanisms to manage emotions, reduce self-destructive behaviors, and improve relationships.

Outcome: Through consistent participation in DBT, Eva gained significant control over her emotions and impulses. She reported fewer instances of self-harm and improved stability in her relationships.

These case studies showcase the diverse approaches and strategies used in mental health care to address various disorders, emphasizing the importance of personalized treatment plans that cater to the unique needs of each patient.

Lessons learned and best practices in mental health nursing

Mental health nursing is a complex field that requires a delicate balance of empathy, clinical skills, and constant learning. Through their experiences, mental health nurses accumulate valuable lessons and identify best practices that enhance patient care and contribute to better outcomes. Here are some key lessons learned and best practices from the field of mental health nursing:

Lessons Learned in Mental Health Nursing

1. **Holistic Approach Is Crucial**

   - Mental health cannot be isolated from physical health; both are intricately linked. Nurses learn that addressing mental health issues effectively also involves considering physical health conditions, lifestyle factors, and social determinants of health.

2. **Empathy Makes a Difference**

   - Showing genuine empathy is not just about understanding patients' feelings but also about validating their emotions and experiences. This can significantly impact the therapeutic relationship and patient trust.

3. **Flexibility in Care**

   - Mental health symptoms and effective interventions can vary widely between patients, even those with the same diagnosis. Nurses learn that flexibility and adaptability in care plans are key to meeting individual patient needs.

4. **Importance of Communication Skills**

   - Effective communication goes beyond verbal interactions. It includes active listening, being aware of nonverbal cues, and being able to convey complex information in an understandable way. Good communication helps in de-escalating crises and building rapport.

5. **Stigma Continues to Be a Barrier**

   - Nurses witness firsthand how stigma negatively affects patient outcomes, discouraging them from seeking or continuing treatment. Fighting stigma is an ongoing challenge that requires continuous effort from healthcare providers.

Best Practices in Mental Health Nursing

1. **Person-Centered Care**

   - Treat each patient as an individual with unique needs, preferences, and values. Person-centered care involves including patients in their treatment planning and decision-making processes, enhancing their autonomy and engagement in treatment.

2. **Use of Evidence-Based Practices**

   - Stay informed about the latest research and clinical guidelines. Using evidence-based practices ensures that the care provided is up-to-date and has the highest chance of being effective.

3. **Continuous Professional Development**

   - Mental health field is always evolving. Regular training and education on new therapies, medications, and care strategies are essential for nurses to remain effective and provide the best care possible.

4. **Safety First**

   - Prioritize safety for patients, staff, and the community. This includes being trained in crisis intervention techniques, understanding when to use de-escalation strategies, and knowing how to apply physical interventions safely if necessary.

5. **Interdisciplinary Collaboration**

- Collaborate with a team of healthcare professionals, including psychiatrists, psychologists, social workers, and occupational therapists. Interdisciplinary teams can provide comprehensive care that addresses all aspects of a patient's health.

6. **Advocacy**

- Advocate for patients' rights and for larger systemic changes that improve mental health care services. This includes pushing for better healthcare policies, more funding for mental health services, and public education to combat stigma.

7. **Support Systems**

- Facilitate connections with community resources, support groups, and other services. Helping patients build a strong support network can greatly improve their recovery and integration into the community.

8. **Reflective Practice**

- Engage in reflective practice regularly. Reflecting on what works well and what doesn't allows nurses to grow

professionally and improve their care
approach continuously.

By integrating these lessons and best practices, mental
health nurses can enhance the quality of care they provide
and make a significant impact on the lives of their patients.
This not only improves patient outcomes but also
contributes to the overall effectiveness and reputation of
the mental health care system.

Interactive questions and reflections on case studies

Here are some examples of interactive questions and
reflective prompts that can be used with mental health
case studies:

Case Study Example

Background: The case study involves "Sarah," a 28-year-
old woman who has been diagnosed with generalized
anxiety disorder (GAD). She struggles with constant worry
about various aspects of her life, such as her job security,
health, and family relationships, which has started to
impair her daily functioning.

Interactive Questions

1. **Assessment Techniques**: What specific techniques
   would you use to assess Sarah's anxiety? How
   would you differentiate her symptoms from other
   possible conditions?

2. **Treatment Planning**: Based on Sarah's symptoms
   of GAD, what initial treatment plan would you
   propose? Consider both pharmacological and non-
   pharmacological interventions.

3. **Patient Education**: How would you explain GAD to Sarah in a way that is both informative and reassuring? What key points would you include about the nature of her disorder and the goals of treatment?

4. **Cultural Considerations**: If Sarah belongs to a cultural group that stigmatizes mental health issues, how would you address this in your treatment approach?

5. **Outcome Evaluation**: What indicators would you look for to assess improvement in Sarah's condition? How might you adjust the treatment plan if the initial interventions are not effective?

Reflection Prompts

1. **Empathy Building**: Reflect on how Sarah might be feeling about her symptoms and diagnosis. How can understanding her perspective help you in providing compassionate care?

2. **Ethical Considerations**: Consider a scenario where Sarah is reluctant to use medication because of perceived stigma. How would you handle this situation ethically, respecting her autonomy while also providing professional guidance?

3. **Professional Development**: Reflect on your own feelings when dealing with patients like Sarah who have anxiety disorders. How can you manage your own stress and maintain a high level of professional care?

4. **Team Collaboration**: Imagine that you are part of a multidisciplinary team managing Sarah's case. What roles would different team members play, and how can effective communication within the team enhance Sarah's care?

5. **Long-term Care Management**: Consider the long-term management of GAD. What strategies would you recommend to Sarah for managing potential relapses or worsening of her symptoms?

Case Study Example

Background: The case involves "Tom", a 34-year-old man recently diagnosed with schizophrenia. He has been experiencing auditory hallucinations and delusional thinking which have disrupted his ability to work and maintain social relationships.

Interactive Questions

1. **Diagnostic Process**: What steps would you take to confirm Tom's diagnosis of schizophrenia? What other conditions might you need to rule out based on his symptoms?

2. **Medication Adherence**: Considering the challenges often associated with medication adherence in schizophrenia, what strategies would you implement to encourage Tom to consistently take his medication?

3. **Therapeutic Approaches**: Besides medication, what psychotherapeutic approaches would be

most appropriate for Tom? How would you integrate these into his overall care plan?

4. **Social Support**: How would you involve Tom's family or support system in his care? What information would you provide to them about schizophrenia?

5. **Crisis Management**: If Tom expresses thoughts of self-harm or shows signs of a severe psychotic episode, what immediate actions would you take?

Reflection Prompts

1. **Understanding Psychosis**: Reflect on the challenges Tom faces in differentiating between reality and his delusions or hallucinations. How might this insight affect your approach to communicating with him?

2. **Stigma and Social Perception**: Consider how societal perceptions of schizophrenia might affect Tom. How could you advocate for Tom in both the healthcare system and his community to help reduce stigma?

3. **Professional Responsibility**: Reflect on your role as a mental health nurse in managing a complex case like schizophrenia. What are the key aspects of providing holistic care for someone with this diagnosis?

4. **Interprofessional Collaboration**: Imagine collaborating with a psychiatrist, a social worker, and a psychologist on Tom's case. What unique

contributions would each professional make, and how can you ensure cohesive care?

5. **Long-term Considerations**: Think about the long-term goals for Tom's treatment. What would successful management of his condition look like, and how can you help him work towards these goals?

These interactive questions and reflection prompts are designed to encourage a deeper exploration of the complexities involved in managing schizophrenia and similar mental health conditions. By engaging with these scenarios, participants can develop a more nuanced understanding of mental health challenges and refine their approaches to patient care, ultimately leading to better patient outcomes.

Using these interactive questions and reflection prompts can enhance learning and engagement during case study discussions, providing learners with a deeper understanding of mental health conditions and the complexities of providing care. This approach not only bolsters clinical skills but also prepares mental health professionals to handle the emotional and ethical dimensions of their work more effectively.

Appendices

Glossary of terms used in mental health nursing

1. **Affective Disorders**: Disorders characterized by changes in mood or affect, typically depression or bipolar disorder.

2. **Anhedonia**: Loss of interest in and withdrawal from all regular and pleasurable activities.

3. **Antidepressants**: Medications used to treat depressive disorders and sometimes other conditions.

4. **Antipsychotics**: Medications used to manage psychosis, including delusions, hallucinations, and disordered thinking.

5. **Anxiety Disorders**: A group of mental health disorders characterized by significant feelings of anxiety and fear.

6. **Behavioral Therapy**: A type of psychotherapy that aims to change potentially self-destructing behaviors.

7. **Bipolar Disorder**: A mental health condition marked by extreme mood swings from highs (mania or hypomania) to lows (depression).

8. **Case Management**: A collaborative process to plan, seek, advocate for, and monitor services from different social services or health care providers.

9. **Cognitive Behavioral Therapy (CBT)**: A psychotherapeutic approach that addresses dysfunctional emotions, behaviors, and cognitions through a goal-oriented, systematic process.

10. **Comorbidity**: The presence of one or more additional diseases or disorders co-occurring with a primary disease or disorder.

11. **Crisis Intervention**: Immediate, short-term help to individuals who experience an event that produces emotional, mental, physical, and behavioral distress.

12. **Delusions**: Strong beliefs that are inconsistent with reality, despite evidence to the contrary.

13. **Dementia**: A chronic or persistent disorder of the mental processes caused by brain disease or injury and marked by memory disorders, personality changes, and impaired reasoning.

14. **Depression**: A mood disorder that causes a persistent feeling of sadness and loss of interest.

15. **Diagnosis**: The identification of the nature and cause of anything. In health care, the term is generally used to identify a disease or disorder.

16. **DSM-5 (Diagnostic and Statistical Manual of Mental Disorders, Fifth Edition)**: The 2013 update to the American Psychiatric Association's classification and diagnostic tool.

17. **Dual Diagnosis**: The coexistence of both a mental health and a substance use disorder.

18. **Eating Disorders**: Mental disorders defined by abnormal eating habits that negatively affect a person's physical or mental health.

19. **Efficacy**: The ability to produce a desired or intended result.

20. **Empathy**: The ability to understand and share the feelings of another.

21. **Ethics**: Moral principles that govern a person's behavior or the conducting of an activity.

22. **Evidence-Based Practice**: Clinical decision-making based on the best available scientific evidence.

23. **Hallucinations**: Experience involving the apparent perception of something not present.

24. **HIPAA (Health Insurance Portability and Accountability Act)**: United States legislation that provides data privacy and security provisions for safeguarding medical information.

25. **Informed Consent**: A process for getting permission before conducting a healthcare intervention on a person.

26. **Intervention**: The act of intervening, interfering or interceding with the intent of modifying the outcome.

27. **Mania**: A mental state of elevated mood, arousal, and energy level.

28. **Mental Health**: A level of psychological well-being, or an absence of mental illness.

29. **Mood Disorders**: Psychological disorders characterized by the elevation or lowering of a person's mood, such as depression or bipolar disorder.

30. **Neurosis**: A class of functional mental disorders involving distress but neither delusions nor hallucinations.

31. **Neurotransmitters**: Chemicals that transmit signals across a synapse from one neuron (brain cell) to another 'target' neuron.

32. **Non-compliance**: Failure or refusal to comply with something (such as a rule or regulation).

33. **Obsessive-Compulsive Disorder (OCD)**: An anxiety disorder characterized by intrusive thoughts that produce uneasiness, apprehension, fear, or worry; by repetitive behaviors aimed at reducing the associated anxiety.

34. **Panic Disorder**: An anxiety disorder characterized by recurrent unexpected panic attacks.

35. **Patient Advocacy**: Various actions aimed to identify and fulfill the needs and interests of patients.

36. **Pharmacotherapy**: The treatment of disease through the administration of drugs.

37. **Post-Traumatic Stress Disorder (PTSD)**: A disorder characterized by failure to recover after experiencing or witnessing a terrifying event.

38. **Psychoeducation**: Education supplied to individuals diagnosed with a psychological disorder that emphasizes and supports the understanding of disorders and the development of coping strategies.

39. **Psychopathology**: The study of abnormal behavior and psychological dysfunction.

40. **Psychotherapy**: The treatment of mental disorder by psychological rather than medical means.

41. **Recovery**: A process of change through which individuals improve their health and wellness, live self-directed lives, and strive to reach their full potential.

42. **Relapse**: The recurrence of disease or ill-health behavior.

43. **Resilience**: The capacity to recover quickly from difficulties.

44. **Schizophrenia**: A long-term mental disorder involving a breakdown in the relation between thought, emotion, and behavior, leading to faulty perception, inappropriate actions and feelings,

withdrawal from reality into fantasy and delusion, and a sense of mental fragmentation.

45. **Self-Harm**: Deliberate injury to oneself, typically as a manifestation of a psychological or psychiatric disorder.

46. **Social Anxiety Disorder**: A chronic mental health condition in which social interactions cause irrational anxiety.

47. **Stigma**: A mark of disgrace associated with a particular circumstance, quality, or person.

48. **Substance Use Disorders**: Conditions in which the use of one or more substances leads to a clinically significant impairment or distress.

49. **Suicide**: The act of intentionally causing one's own death.

50. **Support Groups**: Groups of people with common experiences or concerns who provide each other with encouragement, comfort, and advice.

51. **Therapeutic Alliance**: The relationship between a healthcare provider and a patient.

52. **Therapeutic Communication**: Techniques used by health care professionals to support a patient, both verbally and nonverbally.

53. **Treatment Plan**: A detailed plan tailored to an individual patient and includes goals for treatment, specifics of treatment, and a time frame.

54. **Wellness**: The state of being in good health, especially as an actively pursued goal.

55. **Withdrawal Symptoms**: Symptoms that occur after chronic use of a drug is reduced or stopped abruptly.

56. **Wraparound Services**: Intensive, individualized care management process for individuals with serious or complex needs.

57. **Mental Capacity**: The ability to make one's own decisions.

58. **Behavioral Activation**: A technique in psychotherapy that seeks to ameliorate depression through increased contact with positively reinforcing activities.

59. **Cognitive Restructuring**: A core part of Cognitive Behavioral Therapy (CBT) intended to change patterns of thinking or behavior that are behind people's difficulties, and so change the way they feel.

60. **Dialectical Behavior Therapy (DBT)**: A comprehensive mental health and substance abuse treatment program whose ultimate goal is to aid patients in their efforts to build a life worth living.

Resources for further reading and support

Books

1. **"Psychiatric-Mental Health Nursing" by Sheila L. Videbeck** - Provides a solid foundation in psychiatric nursing and includes patient scenarios to illustrate the application of theory to practice.

2. **"Varcarolis' Foundations of Psychiatric Mental Health Nursing: A Clinical Approach" by Margaret Jordan Halter** - A comprehensive guide that includes detailed information on disorders, treatment plans, and case studies.

3. **"Mental Health in Nursing: Theory and Practice for Clinical Settings" by Barry and Harrison** - This book offers a detailed exploration of mental health issues within nursing practice contexts.

Journals

1. **Journal of Psychiatric and Mental Health Nursing** - Offers articles on the latest research and developments in the field.

2. **Archives of Psychiatric Nursing** - Disseminates original, peer-reviewed research crucial for practicing nurses.

3. **Mental Health Practice** - Provides a wide range of information including clinical articles, career features, and legal updates.

Websites

1. **National Institute of Mental Health (NIMH) -** website - Offers a wealth of information on various mental health disorders, including the latest research and clinical trials.

2. **American Psychiatric Nurses Association (APNA) -** website - A professional organization committed to the specialty practice of psychiatric-mental health nursing and wellness promotion.

3. **World Health Organization (WHO) Mental Health -** website - Provides global resources, reports, and updates on mental health policies and practices.

Online Courses and Workshops

1. **Psychiatric-Mental Health Nurse Practitioner Certification Review -** This online course available on various educational platforms like Udemy prepares nurses for certification exams and provides a comprehensive review of psychiatric nursing.

2. **Mental Health First Aid -** Offers training courses that teach how to help someone who is developing a mental health problem or experiencing a mental health crisis.

Support Groups and Forums

1. **National Alliance on Mental Illness (NAMI) -** website - Offers support groups, education, and advocacy for individuals and families dealing with mental illness.

2. **Mental Health America (MHA)** - website - Provides various resources, including tools for early identification of mental health issues and information on living a healthy lifestyle.

Mobile Apps

1. **Moodfit** - Provides tools to help understand and improve your mental health.

2. **Calm** - Offers meditation and relaxation techniques which can be a beneficial tool for both mental health professionals and their patients to manage stress.

Social Media Platforms

1. **The Mighty** - A digital health community created to empower and connect people facing health challenges and disabilities.

2. **Headspace** on YouTube - Provides guided meditations and mindfulness practices that can be beneficial for mental wellness.

Professional organizations for mental health nursing

Professional organizations play a crucial role in supporting mental health nurses by offering resources for education, networking, advocacy, and professional development. Membership in these organizations can provide mental health nurses with the tools and connections necessary to advance their careers and improve their practice. Here are some key professional organizations for mental health nursing:

1. American Psychiatric Nurses Association (APNA)

- **Website**: APNA

- **About**: APNA is a professional organization dedicated to the specialty practice of psychiatric-mental health nursing and wellness promotion, prevention of mental health problems, and the care and treatment of persons with psychiatric disorders. The association offers a wide range of resources including continuing education, a career center, and certification information.

2. International Society of Psychiatric-Mental Health Nurses (ISPN)

- **Website**: ISPN

- **About**: ISPN is an organization that advocates for mental health care, education, and policy worldwide. It supports advanced practice psychiatric-mental health nurses with education opportunities, an annual conference, and a focus on global mental health.

3. Mental Health Nurses Association (MHNA)

- **Website**: Not specific to one region as many countries have their own MHNA-like organizations.

- **About**: This type of organization typically supports mental health nursing professionals through training sessions, conferences, and resources to promote excellence in mental health care.

4. Canadian Federation of Mental Health Nurses (CFMHN)

- **Website**: CFMHN

- **About**: CFMHN is an association of professional psychiatric nurses in Canada, promoting mental health nursing and focusing on the professional needs of its members through advocacy, education, and networking.

5. Royal College of Nursing Mental Health Forum (RCN)

- **Website**: RCN Mental Health Forum

- **About**: Based in the UK, this forum within the Royal College of Nursing offers resources and discussion platforms for nurses involved in mental health care. It provides guidance, latest updates in practice, and advocacy for mental health issues.

6. Australian College of Mental Health Nurses (ACMHN)

- **Website**: ACMHN

- **About**: ACMHN is the peak professional mental health nursing organization in Australia, which provides standards for practice, education, research, and advocacy in mental health nursing.

7. American Association of Nurse Practitioners (AANP)

- **Website**: AANP

- **About**: While not exclusively for mental health, AANP supports nurse practitioners in all specialties, including psychiatric-mental health. They offer resources such as professional development, practice information, advocacy, and patient education materials.

Benefits of Membership

Joining these organizations can offer several benefits, including:

- **Networking Opportunities**: Connect with peers and leaders in the field for support and career advancement.

- **Continuing Education and Professional Development**: Access to courses, webinars, conferences, and certification programs that help nurses stay at the forefront of their specialty.

- **Advocacy and Influence**: Participate in shaping public policy and advocacy efforts related to mental health nursing and healthcare.

- **Research and Best Practices**: Stay updated with the latest research and best practices in mental health nursing.

Membership in these organizations supports not only individual professional growth but also the broader goal of improving mental health care standards and policies worldwide.

References

Beck, C. T. (2020). "A meta-synthesis of qualitative research on postpartum depression." International Journal of Nursing Studies, 104, 103527.

Relevance: Offers deep insights into the qualitative experiences of postpartum depression, useful for understanding patient perspectives in mental health nursing.

Cleary, M., Raeburn, T., & Escott, P. (2015). "An examination of environmental influences on the well-being of healthcare workers." International Journal of Mental Health Nursing, 24(3), 253-260.

Relevance: Discusses the impact of workplace environments on mental health nurses' well-being, important for understanding the challenges in the profession.

Kisely, S., Abajobir, A. A., Mills, R., Strathearn, L., Clavarino, A., & Najman, J. M. (2020). "Child maltreatment and mental health problems in adulthood: birth cohort study." The British Journal of Psychiatry, 217(6), 674-679.

Relevance: Highlights long-term mental health outcomes of early life experiences, informing psychiatric nursing practices.

Ng, Q. X., Lim, D. Y., & Chee, K. T. (2021). "Managing depression in primary care." Journal of General Internal Medicine, 36(8), 2587-2593.

Relevance: Provides practical guidelines for the management of depression in non-specialist settings, useful for mental health nurses working in community and primary care settings.

Sampaio, F., Sequeira, C., & Teixeira, L. (2018). "Nurses' mental health: the impact of stress and burnout." Industrial Health, 56(5), 450-458.

Relevance: Examines factors contributing to mental health issues among nurses themselves, a critical aspect of nursing education and self-care.

Lakeman, R., & FitzGerald, M. (2008). "How people live with or get over being suicidal: a review of qualitative studies." Journal of Advanced Nursing, 64(2), 114-126.

Relevance: Offers insight into the recovery process from suicidality, pertinent for mental health nursing interventions.

www.ingramcontent.com/pod-product-compliance
Lightning Source LLC
Chambersburg PA
CBHW070756290326
41931CB00011BA/2040